Teaching Clinical Nursing

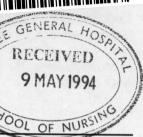

Edited by

Susan M. Hinchliff

B.A., S.R.N., R.N.T.
Formerly Senior Lecturer in Nursing Studies,
Polytechnic of the South Bank, London.
Visiting Lecturer, Polytechnic of the South Bank
and Royal College of Nursing, London.
Academic Editor, Distance Learning Centre,
Polytechnic of the South Bank, London

SECOND EDITION

CHURCHILL LIVINGSTONE
EDINBURGH LONDON MELBOURNE AND NEW YORK 1986

CHURCHILL LIVINGSTONE
Medical Division of Longman Group UK Limited

Distributed in the United States of America by
Longman Inc., 1560 Broadway, New York, N.Y.
10036, and by associated companies, branches and
representatives throughout the world.

First edition 1979
Second edition 1986

ISBN 0 443 02845 1

British Library Cataloguing in Publication Data
Teaching clinical nursing. – 2nd ed.
  1. Nursing – Study and teaching
  I. Hinchliff, Susan M.
  610.73'07'11   RT71

Library of Congress Cataloging-in-Publication Data
Main entry under title:
Teaching clinical nursing.
  Includes index.
  1. Nursing – Study and teaching. 2. Medicine,
Clinical – Study and teaching. I. Hinchliff, Susan M.
[DNLM: 1. Education, Nursing – Great Britain.
2. Teaching. WY 18 T2515]
RT71.T33   1986   610.73'07'11   85-32550

Produced by Longman Singapore Publishers (Pte) Ltd
Printed in Singapore.

Preface to Second Edition

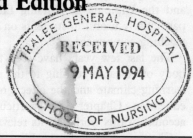

This second edition of *Teaching Clinical Nursing* represents a considerable expansion on the approach and material included in the first edition.

The need to alter existing text in every chapter, and to include new information and ideas, has been brought about by the changes in nursing and nurse education since the first edition.

During that time, the nursing process (or, for those who prefer it, the delivery of individualised nursing care) has become a reality in the majority of hospitals throughout the United Kingdom. Its underlying principles provide a foundation for the ways in which student nurses are currently educated. It has therefore been the aim throughout this entire edition to emphasise the need to teach the art and science of nursing using a problem-solving approach – that is, an approach which underlies the assessment, planning, delivery and evaluative stages of individualised nursing care.

A recent major change in nursing throughout the UK has been the inception of the United Kingdom Central Council for Nursing, Midwifery and Health Visiting (UKCC), together with the four National Boards, which took over their duties from the original statutory bodies on 1 July 1983.

This edition has been able to take account of some changes already wrought by the new structure (e.g. the move towards changing the designated titles for qualified nurses, the incorporation of the JBCNS into the English National Board), but doubtless any future editions will need radical alterations to incorporate further changes.

In the last six years, nursing education has had to adjust to the needs for change in nurse training imposed by the EEC directives; details of these, where relevant, are included in the text.

In the sphere of post-registration nurse education, two major changes that have occurred have been the revisions to the courses offered by certain institutions of further and higher education validated by the University of London – the Diploma in Nursing and the Diploma in Nursing Education. This edition should be particularly useful to students on the latter course, with its clinical teaching component.

The last few years have seen the publication of a considerable body of research relating to the role of the ward sister, the ward learning climate and the effects of both on patient care and nurse education. Chapter 3, in particular, has been expanded to take account of this work and its relevance to teaching clinical nursing.

Chapters 4 and 5 have been revised to include more material specifically related to learning theories appropriate to nurse education, together with increased information on the learning of skills and problem-solving in nursing. This latter topic receives further treatment in Chapter 6, where in addition the theme of the learner as a resource person is further developed.

Throughout 1982 and 1983, the National Health Service underwent a phase of restructuring, with the disappearance of the area health authorities. This has meant regrading of personnel throughout the entire service. At the present time, there appears to be no clear designation for the grade of nurse manager in line above the grade of ward sister. In some authorities, the designation of Nursing Officer has been retained; in others, the term Senior Nurse is used. These two terms have therefore been used interchangeably throughout this book.

In conclusion, when one considers the changes that have occurred in the last few years within the nursing profession (and hence the changes that have become necessary in this edition), it is perhaps salutary to consider the words of Edmund Burke: 'A state without the means of some change is without the means of its conservation'.

St Albans 1986   S. M. H.

Preface to First Edition

The nurse training programme in the United Kingdom has traditionally been run along the lines of an apprenticeship system.

Student nurses have been taught the theory of their art, craft or profession (call it what you will) by their tutors in the school of nursing, and they have learned the practice of their skills at the patient's bedside.

If they were very lucky, they learned their skills at the hands of their tutors, clinical teachers and ward sisters, but frequently the knowledge was passed on by other student nurses, slightly more senior in terms of training or experience on that particular ward.

Learning was often a hit or miss affair, and very much by trial and error. Information was purveyed by these more senior nurses, who were unfamiliar with teaching skills and whose motivation to teach came largely from the fact that a job needed to be done. Times have changed. Student nurses today have the benefit of tutors working in the wards alongside them; they also have ward tutorials, an expansion in the number of clinical teachers and a better planned system of nurse education, with theory related to practice.

This book is written for all nurses who teach in the clinical situation, i.e. where the patient is – whether they are already qualified as nurse teachers, training to become nurse teachers, or are simply interested in teaching in order to support their main work of clinical nursing.

It is not intended as an academic treatise, but rather as a book which sets out to give practical help with the task of teaching.

I can think of no better summary than that given by Florence Nightingale in her preface to *Notes on Nursing*: 'I do not pretend to teach her how, I ask her to teach herself, and for this purpose I venture to give her some hints'.

1978   S. M. H.

Contributors

Elizabeth J. Ballantyne S.R.N., R.S.C.N., S.C.M., D.N., R.C.N.T., MSc.
Formerly Senior Nurse, Research, West Lambeth Health Authority, London

Patricia Boaden S.R.N., D.N., H.V., H.V.T., F.W.T.
Formerly Lecturer in Health Visiting, Polytechnic of the South Bank, London

Barbara Bowron B.A., S.R.N., R.M.N., R.N.T.
Principal Lecturer in Nursing Studies, Polytechnic of the South Bank, London

Mary Chapple M.Ed., S.R.N., D.N., R.C.N.T., R.N.T.
Senior Lecturer in Nursing Studies, Polytechnic of the South Bank, London

Janet Clark B.Ed., S.R.N., D.N., R.C.N.T., R.N.T.
Senior Nurse Tutor, Bristol and Weston School of Nursing, Bristol

Lesley Munro S.R.N., D.N., R.C.N.T., R.N.T., B.Ed.
Senior Lecturer in Nursing Studies, Garnett College, London

Susan M. Hinchliff B.A., S.R.N., R.N.T.
Formerly Senior Lecturer in Nursing Studies, Polytechnic of the South Bank. Visiting Lecturer, Polytechnic of South Bank and Royal College of Nursing, London

Allwyn Holding R.S.C.N., S.R.N., S.C.M.
Formerly Paediatric Ward Sister, The Middlesex Hospital, London

Philippa McMillan S.R.N., R.S.C.N., R.C.N.T., D.N.
Formerly Clinical Teacher, The Middlesex Hospital, London

Ellen Perry B.A., S.R.N., S.C.M., R.N.T., F.R.C.N.
Formerly Principal Lecturer in Nursing Studies, Polytechnic of the South Bank, London

Gordon Rose Ac. Dip. Ed., Cert. Ed., Dip. Special Ed.
Formerly Senior Lecturer in Education, Polytechnic of the South
Bank, London

Contents

Editor's introduction

It seemed particularly timely that, as I prepared to edit this second edition with its revised material, the Report of the Working Party on the Preparation and Education of Nurse Teachers should be published by the Royal College of Nursing.

In my Introduction to the first edition of *Teaching Clinical Nursing*, I cited the recommendations of the Working Party report *The Teachers of Nursing – 1976* published by the General Nursing Council for England and Wales. Briefly, this report urged that:

1. For the learners, the strands of learning should be inextricably intertwined in terms of attitudes, knowledge and skills, in order to carry out the nursing process;
2. Much more emphasis should be placed on preparing ward sisters and all trained staff for their contribution to training in their wards;
3. Entry to the teaching side of the profession should be by a single portal, and nurse teachers should be prepared to teach both in the clinical and classroom settings.

Nine years later, as I suggested in my Preface to the Second Edition, we have gone some way towards meeting the first recommendation. The second and third recommendations, though, are still central issues in the Report of the Rcn Working Party.

The Working Party considered that professional nursing activity fell into a number of definable roles, each of which needed planned preparation for its effective discharge. They considered, in particular, five definable roles pertaining to the teaching of nursing and nurse education:

1. 'The management of nursing within a clinical setting (microenvironment) conducive to the learning of nursing'

This role was seen as being that of the ward sister, and the recent

1

nursing research detailed in Chapter 3 of this edition is crucial to its effective discharge.

2. 'The teaching of nursing practice within clinical environments'

The members of the Working Party felt that it was 'quite wrong to restrict the teaching of nursing practice within clinical environments by grade', and envisaged that the ward sister, the clinical teacher and the nurse tutor would all play a part in this, following adequate preparation and education.

3. 'The teaching of a knowledge-base for nursing within non-clinical environments'

It was felt that 'the teaching of nursing knowledge applied to nursing practice, and based upon the individual's own experience, is likely to be the most effective approach to communicating knowledge, skills and attitudes to those learning to nurse'. This implies the need for continuing sound experience in clinical nursing and hence the marriage of the second and third roles.

4. 'The management of educational processes, particularly curriculum development, and the establishment of macroenvironments conducive to education'

5. 'The management of institutions of nursing education'

On the basis of the identification of these five major roles pertaining to nurse education, the Working Party made certain recommendations, some of which I list below.

In respect of the first three roles (and it is these with which this book is principally concerned), their recommendations were that:

a. 'All ward sisters should have extensive preparation to undertake their roles. This preparation should include extension of their knowledge base in nursing and the development of communication and teaching skills.'

This recommendation is broadly in line with the views of the UKCC regarding continuing education for qualified nurses.

b. 'All courses for nurse teachers should prepare them to teach nursing practice within clinical environments, and the knowledge base for nursing within non-clinical environments.'

c. 'There should be one grade of nurse teacher' while

d. protecting the employment status of those currently qualified as clinical teachers.

e. 'Nurse teachers should be required to maintain and develop clinical nursing skills appropriate to the area of nursing they will teach, and have the opportunity to do so'.

These are welcome proposals, and it is the stated policy of the Rcn to 'endeavour to influence the profession and the relevant authorities to take steps to implement the recommendations'. It is to be hoped, therefore, that the next edition of this book will be able to report the fulfilment of this aim.

From the foregoing, it is evident that nurse tutors (many of whose experience to date may have provided them with restricted opportunities for clinical teaching), staff nurses and ward sisters will all need guidance in developing, or updating their teaching skills in the ward setting.

This book, whose contributors are all concerned with nurse education, aims to help in a practical way anyone who has to teach nursing in the ward, specialised unit or community. The subjects covered range from nursing itself (what it *is* and a little of what it *should* be); the role of the clinical teacher; opportunities for ward teaching, given the real problems that are encountered and how the teacher learns to cope with them; a brief review of some educational theories underpinning teaching techniques; on a practical note, there is a chapter on teaching aids and resources; a consideration of clinical teaching in various settings, *viz.* the psychiatric unit, the paediatric unit, the community and the setting up of post-basic courses in specialised units (all of which call for modification in teaching techniques from the general approach discussed earlier); and, finally, a discussion of the developing role of the clinical teacher, tracing this from the 1930s to the present day.

There is emphasis throughout the book on the development of skills required for good clinical teaching: for instance, observation, communication, human relationships, problem-solving, working as a team with other professionals, specifying clear objectives, and integrating theory and practice – to name but a few.

As well as the traditional index, a glossary of terms used in the text has been compiled. This should be useful in providing brief definitions of some of the concepts referred to by contributors.

In the interests of brevity, the words 'she' and 'her' have been used to refer to any nurse, whether male or female; the term 'ward sister' implies any person in charge of a ward; and 'student' is used in its broadest sense to denote any nurse in training.

Finally, perhaps, I should state, that my aim in compiling this work is that those who teach in the clinical setting should develop a very real enjoyment of the task. I hope that this book will prove helpful.

REFERENCES

General Nursing Council for England and Wales 1976 The Teachers of Nursing Report of the R.C.N. Working Party 1983. The Preparation and Education of Teachers of Nursing. London: Royal College of Nursing.

1

The process of clinical nursing

If you have read the preface, you will have read that this is a book which sets out to give some practical help with the task of teaching nursing. You may therefore be wondering why the book starts off with a chapter on nursing itself.

Surely, you may ask, once you come to teach a subject, can it not be assumed that you already have a sufficient grasp of the content to be taught?

To a certain extent, this is an assumption that is implicit in many of the courses available in this country at the moment to those who wish to learn how to teach nursing. In order to obtain a certificate or diploma in nurse education, it is not always necessary to further one's knowledge of the art and science of nursing as a discipline in itself.

I do not feel that this a valid assumption. One has never finished learning about nursing or furthering one's knowledge in this field, and there have been many relevant recent advances.

If one looks carefully at the nursing curriculum as it was taught in the past, there was little emphasis on nursing as a discipline with a sound scientific basis and its own body of knowledge. There was plenty of emphasis, however, on how nursing measures could support medical measures, and on the motor skills involved in, for instance, changing a dressing or performing specific tasks.

Thus, historically, there was much emphasis on aspects of nursing which contribute towards the whole, but little emphasis on the total caring picture. I am reminded of when I was myself a ward sister on a female medical ward some years ago. At the time, when patients died, I felt that I coped reasonably efficiently with the dying patient, death itself, the bereaved relatives, the administrative and nursing minutiae of the situation, and the necessary practical skills required. It was only when I undertook the Sister Tutor's Diploma and had the privilege of hearing a speaker from St Christopher's Hospice that I realised all the things I had left undone, and all the caring aspects that I could have performed better. I do not think that I was alone in holding those feelings.

That brought home to me how sad it can be to recognise a patient's needs too late, and to fail to give care tailor-made to a particular patient in a particular situation.

What follows is therefore a personal account of the process of clinical nursing. In discussing nursing, firstly one ought to define *what nursing is*.

In many ways, it is easier to explain what it comprises, and what it involves, rather than saying what it *is*.

There have been many attempts at definition; but one that I find useful, albeit somewhat imprecise, is that nursing is 'a caring art based on individual needs'. I shall come back to that later.

Nursing can be said to be made up of a system of skills which are of two main kinds, namely technical and caring.

The technical skills in nursing are often of great complexity – e.g. the management of peritoneal dialysis, intermittent positive pressure ventilation, etc., but may equally be of a relatively simple nature – e.g. taking a temperature or giving an injection.

Traditionally in this country under a task-allocation system of nursing, the more senior one became as a student nurse, the more complex were the technical tasks assigned. Thus, the technical aspects became associated with seniority and experience, and assumed a sort of prestige value. This was in contrast to the more lowly round of blanket baths and bedpans assigned to the more junior exponents of nursing.

These technical skills have an associated theory and a scientific infrastructure, and the importance of learning them was, in the past, underlined by their presence in the student's record of practical experience. Possession of the necessary skill was traditionally therein recorded, and this tended to emphasise technical skill acquisition as providing the milestones in the nurse's experience.

What, though, of the caring aspect of nursing skills? What is the nurse caring about? The caring involves a person who has a health problem, or many problems, which provide the reason for his being in contact with the nurse.

Essentially, caring involves an *individual* who has a family, friends, an occupation, interests, attitudes, values, beliefs, and so on. Good nursing care has always been characterised by the attention paid to meeting the needs of the individual patient. Today we are entering an era in which it is a foremost and explicit aim of nurse educationalists and nurse practitioners to maximise the individualised care delivered to each patient. This chapter seeks to give an outline of how this might be achieved.

When a patient comes into hospital, what do we do first of all? We assign him to a bed with a number; he is given case notes with another number; we take away his clothes and strip him thereby of a certain amount of dignity. We certainly strip him of privacy and of his belongings.

Further, we categorise him and tend to assume that he has feelings and needs appropriate to the category assigned to him. He may be labelled using one of several parameters, e.g. the *amputee* (referring to what we have done to him), the *appendicitis* (referring to the medical condition he has), the *down and out* (referring to his social status), the *West Indian* (referring to his race), the *Jew* (referring to his religion), the *attention-seeker* (referring to his behaviour), the *wealthy patient* (referring to his economic status), the *accountant* (referring to his occupation), the *widower* (referring to his marital status), the *old man* (referring to his age), the *patient in bed ten* (referring to his ward position).

I am sure most nurses have used these labels at some time. Indeed, they can be useful, provided that they are used to *fill out* a total picture of an individual, and provided that they are not used in isolation to describe the total patient.

Having said this, I turn now to *what caring involves*. First of all, it involves giving. In order to nurse a patient well, one has to give of oneself to him, often to the extent that one feels drained after caring for the patient. One gives love, understanding, compassion; one empathises; and one gives respect, thereby giving back to the patient some of the dignity and worth of which he feels stripped.

Traditionally, student nurses were warned against becoming too attached to a patient. Detachment from over-involvement was seen as a state to aim for. However, very few of the student nurses I have worked with have remained truly detached in the face of death, pain, injury or disfigurement; and indeed nowadays one would question whether such a state were desirable.

Perhaps one should put oneself on the position of the young parents whose only child has just died of leukaemia. Their need is for a nurse who cares for them, cares about the death of their child, and who remains calm and supportive. But do they really appreciate a totally flattened emotional response? I think not. Caring involves recognition that one is involved.

Caring also involves giving both physical and psychological support. Nursing used to have a 'cool hands on fevered brow' image; subsequently, there was a swing away from this in favour of the unglamorous hardworking image. I am not sure that we have not swung too far away from the former approach. A fan is a very efficient agent for lowering temperature, but it is the cool hand that assures the patient that there is someone there who cares.

Caring involves sharing. When John Donne said that 'No man is an *Island*, entire of itself', he was not speaking in the context of a hospital ward, but his words are particularly apt in that situation. Nursing means sharing the triumphs; sharing the sense of achievement when the aphasic patient after a cerebrovascular accident manages to ask clearly for a drink; sharing the first steps of the arthritic patient after a total hip replacement; sharing the joy of the patient discharged after a heart operation. It also means sharing the grief and the pain; sharing the sadness of the woman who has once more aborted a longed-for fetus; sharing the phantom limb pains of the patient who has had a leg amputated; sharing the desperation of the young man with cancer.

In the latter cases, caring also involves giving hope along with support. One can support the patient technically; one can also support by simply being there, by touching, by listening and by well-chosen words. Often, in the case of the terminally ill patient, the hope that one can give is restricted to the hope for relief from pain, or for a peaceful and dignified death.

Caring involves giving knowledge; thus, it involves teaching the patient to cope unaided once the nursing support is withdrawn. However good, the nursing care of the newly diabetic patient is as nothing if we do not extent his competence so that he can cope with his disability himself once he is discharged from our care.

Often, caring just means being there while the patient learns for himself what he can and cannot now do. It is not caring to protect the patient to the extent that he cannot survive without the nurse.

To care implies that a need for care exists on the part of the patient. The fact that one is needed provides a large degree of job satisfaction to most nurses; it is, however, important that the nurse does not set out to satisfy her need to be needed, at the expense of the patient once he has progressed beyond being a passive recipient.

Caring may involve concealing. It may involve concealing our dislike of a particular patient. A nurse cannot hope to like all of her patients equally, and her realisation of this may instil feelings of guilt in her. Nevertheless, this dislike must be concealed. Likewise, she must conceal distaste and revulsion. The junior nurse, seeing mutilation for the first time, or extensive surgical intervention for a disfiguring condition, needs help in caring for the patient, to enable her to conceal her disgust and perhaps fear.

It involves concealing her own lack of hope, which she may feel when nursing the young patient with cancer. As stated before, the nurse needs help to realise that there is always hope, if only for a quiet death. It also involves concealing prejudices.

Caring, finally, involves integrity. It involves adhering to a code of professional conduct which protects the patient from malpractice and negligence. Caring involves more than all of these; total caring is more than the sum of the individual parts to the patient to whom the care is rendered.

To recap, nursing involves two kinds of skills (technical and caring). The combination of these two skills leads to the development of clinical judgement, the possession of which is the sign of a mature nurse: mature in both the professional and the personal sense. Clinical judgement has nothing to do with age, but a lot to do with experience; and it is this quality which one aims to develop in the student nurse.

At this point, I would like to turn to the thoughts of Virginia Henderson (1958) on nursing care. She said:

'The unique function of the nurse is to assist the individual, sick or well, in the performance of those activities contributing to health or its recovery (or to peaceful death) that he would perform unaided if he had the necessary strength, will or knowledge'.

This, to me, describes succinctly what the nurse *does*. She goes on to say what the nurse *is*:

'She is temporarily the consciousness of the unconscious, the love of life for the suicidal, the leg of the amputee, the eyes of the newly blind, a means of locomotion for the infant, knowledge and confidence for the young mother, the mouthpiece for those too weak or withdrawn to speak, and so on'.

This, I think, brings us back to the definition of nursing stated earlier, namely a 'caring art based on individual needs', since the above statements of Virginia Henderson assume the existence of the patient's needs.

Imagine a patient coming into hospital for the first time. He is unfamiliar with the system, and this is a totally new experience. What are his needs?

Firstly, he needs to be understood as an individual, Understanding of a person may take more time than the nurse has at her disposal, but she can make an attempt at this by gathering as much information about him as possible – information that helps her to build up a picture of him as a person.

Some time ago, I had occasion to sit in on a ward teaching session where a clinical teacher was discussing the total care of a man who had had a myocardial infarction. The student nurses she was teaching had an impressive array of facts at their fingertips with regard to the patient's cardiac arrhythmias and enzyme level disturbances. What they were not able to tell the teacher, however, was that the patient's wife had died only four weeks previously. They were competent in their exercise of *technical* skills, but lacking in their *caring* skills, and without this piece of vital information were unable to respond to the patient's needs, or even to define them.

Next, the patient needs information – at a variety of levels. He needs to know more about what is wrong with him and what is going to be done to him. Suddenly, he is no longer in control of the situation – no longer in control, even, of himself and his body image. When malfunction occurs, the patient's perception of himself is impaired, and he is anxious and vulnerable. The information given to a patient may have a marked effect on, for example, his perception of pain and need for analgesia (Hayward 1975), or on his post-operative recovery (Boore 1978).

The previously fit and active businessman, used to holding and delegating authority, suddenly finds himself in pain, unsure of his diagnosis and frightened of the possible outcome. He needs information about the disease, and what the signs and symptoms mean; he needs to know what investigations are likely to be necessary, what therapeutic procedures might be undertaken, how long these will take, what the prognosis might be, and so on.

In hospital, we usually attempt to give the patient information, but it is not always the information *he* needs to know. Too often, it is the information *we* choose to give him, expressed in terms familiar to *us* but foreign to him, and given in amounts that *we* deem suitable, and at times convenient to us.

It is easy to assume, once the patient is told that she has uterine fibroids and that she is to have a hysterectomy, that this is the end of the matter. We assume that she then knows and understands what is happening to her. This is almost always not so. Anxiety and fear tend to cloud understanding, and explanations have to be given with patience – and repeatedly if desired by the patient, although this desire may not be overtly expressed.

The patient needs to feel secure. This is easy to say, but difficult to achieve. Imagine, once more, the patient in hospital for the first time. Hospital is very different from home in every respect. The smells are different, and may be strange or even unpleasant to some patients as may the sights to which the patient is exposed. When a newly admitted patient is frightened and anxious, and then placed in a bed next to a patient who is confused and disorientated, who has an intravenous infusion, a nasogastric tube, and urinary drainage apparatus, all of which are visible, this may do much to worsen the new patient's fears. Intimations of mortality are frequent in hospital, and the hospital staff, so used to these sights, underestimate the anxiety they may instil in new patients.

The noises, too, are strange. To the patient unable to sleep in the dimly lit hospital ward, with its unfamiliar sounds, the bubbling respirations of the patient opposite with chronic bronchitis may be unbelievably frightening and disturbing.

The daily routine in hospital is different from home. The patient may be unused to the hours of rising and lights out. Suddenly, he is no longer able to watch the late news on television. The radios may be turned off at an early hour, and the channels available pre-selected. He is no longer able to get up to the toilet in the night, however able he may feel to do so.

He is surrounded by furniture to which he is unused. The arthritic patient may find that the only available armchair is too low for his comfort. His bed may be too high for easy access. He may not know how to use the lamp, earphones or bell attachments on his locker. He is denuded of his usual comforts and possessions.

The food in hospital is different from that to which he is used. It is served in different amounts, at different times, and may be unpalatable to him.

Simply because he is a patient, he may find that he is put into a wheelchair to go to X-ray department, although he feels perfectly able to walk.

All of these serve further to alter his perception of himself and his abilities. The mores of the hospital are well and truly imposed from above. All of these unfamiliar aspects of hospital life serve to lessen his feelings of security. A well thought-out explanation of the ward routine, on admission, may do much to lessen his fears.

The patient needs reassurance. This is a well recognised fact, but it is easier to talk about than to carry out, however. Perhaps, though, it can be subsumed under several other need headings.

The patient needs to feel accepted. Previous to his admission, the patient has been accepted by his family, friends, colleagues, neighbours, those with whom he is in a service relationship, and so on; but on admission to the hospital he feels somewhat bereft of these supports, and deprived of his familiar group memberships.

Frequently, the patient feels shut off from his family who, feeling that he should not be worried by what is going on at home, exclude him from discussion of domestic problems, exude false cheerfulness, and concentrate at visiting time on discussing the hospital situation, when the patient really needs to feel that he is missed by his family, and not so dispensable as they tend to imply.

He needs to feel accepted, uncritically, by fellow patients, doctors and nurses. He may feel ashamed or embarrassed by his illness, and desperately needs to feel less abnormal.

He needs privacy. At home, he can shut himself away if he needs solitude. This is not possible in hospital. Privacy is needed at several levels. Some time ago, when visiting a relative in hospital, I was horrified to be told that an elderly lady who had had an artificial leg for many years was required to keep her prosthesis at night on a shelf above her bed, as it seemed that the nurses were unable to provide her with a more suitable place for its temporary storage. This was a sight that was traumatic for other patients, and caused the lady herself acute embarrassment and loss of dignity. Thus, privacy is necessary for carrying out intimate personal tasks. It is also necessary for personal discussion.

Imagine the young patient who wishes to discuss with his wife whether he should agree to an operation which would render him impotent. This is not a subject which they can discuss with patients adjacent, perhaps only a few feet away.

It is questionable whether we provide the privacy that patients need, or even attempt to assess the degree of privacy which a particular patient needs.

The patient needs to have confidence in those treating him, confidence that they know what they are doing and know what is best for him. When he sees that the nurses are competent, and that student nurses, albeit learners, are adequately supervised, then he will feel reassured.

The patient needs to know what his role is. Often the new patient has no idea what he is expected, or able, to do in his new *milieu*. Should he get up, or stay in bed, or get dressed, or sit up at the table for meals? He needs to have all of these basic questions answered, as well as questions related to his treatment. He needs to know, for example, that after a total knee replacement his rehabilitation largely depends on his own efforts; only thus can he work towards and derive a sense of achievement from, his own progress.

The patient needs stimulation. I am not suggesting that this has to be intense and tiring, merely that he needs to have some purposeful activity once the stage of acute illness has passed. Such stimulation should be of the patient's own choosing. For instance, jigsaws are all very well if you enjoy them, but are not helpful therapy for those who have developing cataracts or arthritis.

The patient needs to be listened to. After all, the patient may have lived with his disability for some years, and may therefore be in the best position to tell the nurse how he finds it easiest to move. Just by listening intelligently to the patient, the nurse can learn much. Most nurses have a limited subjective experience of pain and disease, and they can do much to enhance their knowledge and clinical judgement simply by listening.

To be thought worthy of being listened to enhances the patient's self-esteem. The elderly lady, telling the story of her teenage years in service, gets an enormous psychological fillip from having her nurse just sit and listen.

The young man, dying of carcinoma, needs to talk about his fears, his fear of the dying process itself, his fears for those he leaves behind, his fears of pain and losing control, his anger at those things he is unable to do, and at the injustice of it all.

The patient's need to talk is often acute, and cannot be fitted into a timetable. When he needs to talk, the nurse needs to listen.

The patient has physical needs: comfort, warmth, freedom from pain, gentleness, rest and peace.

Hay and Anderson (1963), however, analysed patients' needs as expressed to them after the patient had been discharged, and they found that the majority of needs were emotional in nature. They existed in three main areas:

1. The need to have one's identity both recognised and maintained;
2. The need to exercise some control over oneself and one's environment;
3. Needs derived from feelings of fear, anxiety and loneliness.

By now, it should be obvious that the patient has needs; and in order to meet those needs, they must be assessed individually. In the past this assessment was largely intuitive and unstructured. In the last decade, however, in the United Kingdom, there has been a marked attempt to improve the delivery of individualised patient care by providing a framework within which the needs for care can be assessed, a nursing diagnosis formulated, appropriate care can be planned and delivered, and the total care can be evaluated. This framework is sometimes referred to as the nursing process, or individualised care planning.

It is perhaps fitting here to remind ourselves that it was Hippocrates who said 'It is more important to know what sort of person has a disease than to know what sort of disease a person has.' The need for a detailed assessment of the patient clearly did not originate in the United States (as many people think), nor did it become recognised with the advent of the nursing process!

Assessment

Assessment starts with the collection of information about the patient, and ends with the formulation of a nursing diagnosis which allows definition of the patient's problems. It is, essentially, a systematic look at the patient's total behaviour, including physiological, psychological and social aspects, during which the nurse identifies her need to act.

The patient himself

Traditionally in this country, it was the nurse's job to admit the patient. Part of the admission procedure involved the checking and assembly of a body of information usually relating to the patient's age, date of birth, address, religion, occupation, next of kin, etc. This provided a good opportunity to discuss other factors which might impinge on the patient's response to his illness and hospitalisation – for example, finding out if he had been in hospital before, if he would be likely to have any visitors, and so on.

With the introduction of ward receptionists, however, in the early 1960s, it became quite common for the patient to be received and formally admitted by the receptionist, and although the basic information was obtained in an efficient way, many of the small caring points were not elicited. It is currently recognised that the reception and subsequent assessment of the patient is a vital nursing activity, since the care that the nurse will plan for the patient can only be as good as her assessment of the patient allows. If this assessment is perfunctory, then only scant care can be planned; conversely, a detailed assessment allows for comprehensive planning of care.

In order for assessment to be systematic and effective, there are several requirements which merit consideration.

1. Assessment requires a format

This provides a framework or structure which ensures that the information collected at this stage is comprehensive and adequately detailed. Information needs to be collected on several fronts: for example, patients' physical status, the environment from which the patient comes to the hospital, his perception of his health problem and how he responds to it, his degree of role adaptation, his personal habits and the ways in which he normally meets his needs of daily living.

Various models can be used for assessment of the patient, subsequent goal setting and planning of missing care: for example, Virginia Henderson outlined fourteen activities of daily living – sleep, elimination, care of the skin etc – and these provide a measure for the analysis of the patient's activities, allowing the nurse to identify where deficits or needs exist on the part of the patient and hence where care is required on the part of the nurse (Henderson 1966).

A systematic head-to-toe assessment of the patient may be carried out using the Assessment Man (Wolff and Erickson 1977), where the nurse assesses functions – vision, hearing, sensation, etc – and also environmental factors which affect the patient, such as any equipment he needs for daily living.

Another format which may be used is Abdellah's '21 Nursing Problems' model (Abdellah 1960). Abdellah takes 21 aspects (or problems) of nursing care, and the nurse is encouraged to assess the degree to which the patient requires nursing intervention for each problem. Examples of some of Abdellah's problems are:

– to maintain good hygiene and physical comfort;
– to recognise the physiological responses of the body to disease conditions (pathological, physiological and compensatory);
– to identify and accept positive and negative expressions, feelings and reactions.

The model devised by Roper based on Activities of Living is widely accepted in the U.K. and the reader is urged to study this together with a range of other models, such as those proposed by Orem & Roy (see Riehl & Roy 1980).

In other to facilitate assessment, a more or less detailed questionnaire form is commonly used, and this may be referred to as a nursing history. This questionnaire has the advantage of giving some structure to the assessment interview, and so long as open-ended questions are used it allows flexibility. Since the nurse records her initial and subsequent assessments on the form, all the caring team have access to identical information.

The use of a comprehensive form may avoid the situation where the patient often does not volunteer vital information, because he does not perceive it to be important or because he was never asked for it. It also leads to a more objective assessment of the patient's needs.

Perhaps it should be stressed, though, that the questions must be expressed in the patient's language. The questionnaire will not elicit the information required if it is couched in words which the patient does not understand. Neither should it include questions which are phrased in a way which the patient might find offensive; for example, in enquiring about a patient's hygiene arrangements the nurse may wish to know what facilities the patient has for washing at home, and he may respond to this innocent question with some indignation – feeling that the nurse is implying that he is dirty, or that he lives in inadequate housing.

At the same time, while the nurse is observing and questioning she must not reveal by her own facial expressions any distaste or revulsion for what the patient reveals by his words or appearance. She must be non-judgmental in her approach, and must not allow her observations to be tempered by her moods, attitudes or values.

2. Assessment requires privacy

In order to take a nursing history, privacy is necessary. The details which one is to obtain from the patient may be intimate in nature, and he is less likely to divulge information which he may deem embarrassing if he is overlooked or overheard by patients in adjacent beds.

3. Assessment requires skills

a. Observation skills. Much of the information to be gained when assessing the patient comes directly from the personal observations of the nurse.

It was Florence Nightingale (1859) who said:

'the most important practical lesson that can be given to nurses is to teach them what to observe, how to observe, what symptoms indicate improvement and which the reverse, which are of importance and which are of none, which are the evidence of neglect and of what kind of neglect'.

She went on to say:

'if you cannot get the habit of observation one way or another, you had better give up the being of a nurse, for it is not your calling, however kind and anxious you may be'.

The nurse must employ all of her senses in her observations. Her eyes can tell her that the skin looks dry and shrivelled, her touch can tell her that the skin on the back of the hands has lost its elasticity and can be plucked up easily, her sense of smell can tell her that the patient's breath has a faecal taint, her ears can pick up the patient's faint moan. From her senses, she can assess the degree of the patient's dehydration when he is admitted with acute intestinal obstruction.

It should be remembered when trying to help a learner develop observation skills that we often see – that is, perceive — only what we want to see, or what we expect to see. Perception requires prior experience, and if this is lacking then the learner may be unable to observe that which is obvious to the trained nurse. An example of this might be the learner R.M.N. student who is 'tuned in' to observe the degree of anxiety exhibited by the patient, but who may fail to notice the signs which indicate incipient right ventricular failure. Conversely, the student for general training may be so concerned with assessing the degree of jaundice shown by a patient with haemolytic anaemia, that she fails to notice the signs that a patient is becoming severely depressed.

b. Interviewing and listening skills. In order to help the learner develop these skills, the trained nurse may act as a role model and encourage the learner to shadow her while she assesses the patient, thus allowing the student to learn by example and from the subsequent examination of what took place.

Relatives can be a further useful source of information. It may be the patient's wife who reveals that her husband has a dislike of troubling others, and would hesitate to call for analgesia postoperatively, or that he has expressed to her a fear of death, or of having cancer. An interview with the patient's nearest relative or companion may yield much information of value in caring for the patient and may in addition provide support for the relatives.

The nurse can often learn much by developing an awareness of what the patient does *not* say: for example, the question 'Am I going to die?' is often not asked; nevertheless the experienced nurse may perceive that the patient may be troubled and can leave space for the patient gradually to give voice to his anxieties and unspoken fears.

c. Assessment requires measurement skills. In planning care, it is much more valuable to have a measure of the amount of pain experienced by a patient than merely to know that the patient is in pain. Measurement tools have been developed which enable the nurse better to assess various aspects of patients' needs, for example the pain rating scale developed by Hayward (Hayward 1975) and the pressure area assessment scale developed by Norton (Norton 1975).

All of these skills require prior teaching and a great deal of practice before the learner can become proficient in them and in assessment as a whole.

The information gathered at the assessment stage leads to the formulation of a nursing diagnosis, that is, an assessment of the patient's strengths and problems (both actual and potential) based on nursing judgment.

The nursing diagnosis is different from the medical diagnosis. The latter centres on pathology and the resultant signs and symptoms; the nursing diagnosis centres on the effects on the patient of the disease process. For example, the medical diagnosis may be ischaemic heart disease, whereas the nursing diagnosis for the same patient may be shortness of breath on exertion, inability to tolerate the pain which accompanies the disease without extreme agitation, a fear of dying, and so on. The nursing diagnosis may change several times as the patient progresses, and so fear of dying may change to anxiety about coping at home after discharge from hospital.

This assumes, therefore, that nursing assessment must be repeated at planned intervals, and cannot merely be done once and for all on admission. As new problems emerge and initial ones resolve, care must be evaluated and replanned.

The assessment stage of planning individualised patient care calls for both cognitive and intellectual skills; it requires the sorting and classification of information and the interpretation of this against scientific facts and theories, together with the identification of the patient's problems, strengths and needs. Having done this, the nurse is then in a position to plan care for the patient.

Planning care

Ideally, a care plan should be so individualised that it should only be possible to use it for the patient for whom it was designed. This means, therefore, that it should be detailed with respect to all aspects of the particular patient's needs.

At the planning stage, the nurse has all the requisite data, has diagnosed the patient's problems and needs, and is in a position to assign priorities for care. These priorities must coexist with the priorities for care of others in the health team; ideally, therefore, planning should be a multi-disciplinary exercise.

Maslow (1970) envisages a 'pyramid of needs', a hierarchical arrangement with five goals. Only when the lower level needs have been met will the higher level needs emerge into the individual's consciousness. These needs energise the individual towards behaviour designed to meet the needs. This is therefore a theory of motivation for the individual, and hence should be considered by the nurse in planning care.

1. *Physiological needs* from the basis of the pyramid: the needs for food, air, water and so on are of prime importance, and lack of any of these commodities monopolises the consciousness to the extent that there is urgent activity aimed at need satisfaction at this level.
2. *Safety needs* emerge once physiological needs are satisfied. The need for shelter, warmth, avoidance of injury, a secure environment and so on must be met.
3. The need for love (the *affiliation need*) is next in the hierarchy. The individual needs to relate to others in a positive way. He needs to give and to receive love.
4. The *need for esteem and respect* is the next to be realised. The individual has a need to feel worthy of value as a person. He needs to be understood.
5. Finally, at the apex of the pyramid is the *need for self-actualisation* and the need to realise one's potential.

The patient may need to realise a *new* potential, limited by his health problem, and may therefore need help in accepting this.

Perhaps we should ask how often we work towards achieving all five goals; on a busy ward, in dealing with the patient who is perhaps less popular than others, we may only work towards satisfying needs at the bottom two levels, that is, those needs vital for survival. We ensure that the patient has adequate food, fluids, a clear airway, warmth and a comfortable position – but we may sometimes omit to ensure that he feels cared for, respected and capable of realising his full potential.

Maslow's hierarchy of needs should be borne in mind while planning care, and we should work towards gratification at all levels.

The patient himself and those close to him where appropriate should be involved in the planning, and this involvement serves to realise his need for esteem and recognition. The patient with a chronic physical handicap can often be the best person to help plan care with regard to his positioning in bed and mobilisation. Likewise, the arthritic patient can often best advise on meeting his safety needs. It must be remembered, though, that in the end it is the nurse's responsibility, and indeed it may be hers alone when the patient is *in extremis*.

The plan should include not only recognition of present problems and difficulties but should also seek to recognise future problems and complications. It should therefore be a dynamic programme. Care was always planned to a certain degree in nursing, but frequently it was planned on the basis of the medical diagnosis and not around both this and the nursing diagnoses. Planning should provide a creative opportunity: an opportunity for the nurse to exercise her skills in using her clinical judgement. It entails the marriage of theory and clinical expertise, expressing the planner's nursing ideology and philosophy, and it should lead to a prescription for individual care.

An imprecise care plan cannot fail to lead to variations in the care given, depending on who administers it. Florence Nightingale wrote in her *Notes on Nursing*:

'all the results of good nursing, as detailed in these notes, may be spoiled or utterly negatived by one defect, viz. in petty management, or in other words, by not knowing how to manage that what you do when you are there, shall be done when you are not there.'

What better recommendation for the drawing up of a detailed care plan.

One nurse who reads 'fluids plus plus' in the care plan may simply place a jug of water on the patient's locker and give him instructions to drink it. The nurse on the next shift, however, may interpret those words to mean that she should enquire of the patient what he would like to drink and give him 200 ml of the preferred beverage every hour. The patient, faced with this discrepancy in care with regard to his fluid regime, may well feel confused and uncertain as to what he should be doing.

In summary, therefore, a nursing care plan must be practical, taking into consideration the constraints of the ward situation. It must be appropriate to the patient's desires, if possible, as well as to his needs. It must be expressed precisely, and in writing, so that all members of the care team can refer to it. It must include some indication of the priorities allocated to the various aspects of care, and essentially it must be flexible with frequent *reported* revision.

If all these conditions are met, then the time spent in care planning should ultimately save time; time, that is, wasted in asking and answering unnecessary questions. A detailed care plan allows priorities to be set which may save further time if the ward is short-staffed and the nursing staff are busy; under these conditions, the care plan can be used to ensure the patient's safety.

In practical terms, the care plan may take the form of a large chart with three or four columns, each setting out the problem, the goal or objective, the prescribed nursing care, and the method for evaluating this care.

It is useful at this stage to distinguish between goals and objectives. It may seem easier to suggest goals for the patient than to specify objectives. In the case of a patient who has suffered a cerebrovascular accident, it is easy to state that at the end of the caring episode the patient should be in an optimal condition, bearing in mind the constraints with regard to his walking, speech and mental abilities.

Objectives, though, should be more precise; they should describe the expected desired and measurable changes in the patient's behaviour which subserve the long-term goal. They are useful in guiding the nurse's behaviour towards achieving the end goal. For example, long before the hemiplegic patient can walk and feed himself, he should be able to move his limbs a small amount, and put his feet to the ground, bend his knee, put out his hand towards a cup, pick up or grasp it, and so on.

In determining objectives, one needs to set criteria for their achievement. For instance, three weeks after having had a total knee replacement the patient should have 90 degrees of movement in that joint, unaided, without acute pain.

The objectives need to be flexible and tailored to the individual patient; for instance, it might not be possible to achieve the above objective if the patient had needed resuturing of the wound, or had suffered a deep vein thrombosis.

It is obvious at this stage that planning requires the nurse to exercise skills different from those needed at the assessment stage.

Planning requires skills in writing precise and realistic objectives, expressed in measurable and behavioural terms having set achievable goals. For this, clinical experience is necessary, and a broad overview of the possible and probable outcome of treatment.

Planning requires skills in deciding on the actions to be taken to meet defined needs, and an ability to select these from a repertoire of possible nursing activities.

Planning requires skills in deciding how to evaluate such planned nursing activities. Planning is, therefore, not something that can be done by a junior nurse unless she has considerable teaching support and guidance throughout this stage.

The model of nursing care being used for a patient will dictate the actual format and documentation relating to the care plan; however it is likely that whatever the model being used, the following points will be considered:

1. The patient's medical needs: These refer to specific disease-related needs:
   a. Details of the drugs ordered may be included on the care plan: which drug is to be given in which form, how much and how often, times of administration, any precautions to be taken, whether to be given routinely or *pro re nata*;
   b. Investigations with the necessary preparation for treatments to be given should likewise be recorded in this section.
2. Basic physiological bodily needs:
   a. Cleanliness: what type of bath is necessary. Can the patient get up to the bath? If so, can he do so unaided? Should it be a medicated bath? If he is to have a bed bath, how often is this to be performed? This may be related to the patient's general condition or temperature.
   b. The diet should be detailed: whether it is to be a full diet chosen from the ward menu, a light diet prescribed by the dietician, or restricted in terms of calories, proteins, fats, minerals, or enriched in any way with supplements;
   c. The fluids to be taken should be included: how much, of what kinds, how often;

d. Skin care and care of appendages: Does the patient need help with the care of his hair and nails? If so, details should be given. Does he need a chiropodist's attention? Is he able to care for his mouth and teeth himself? Does he have dentures? Does he need help or equipment in caring for his teeth? If he cannot perform mouth care himself, the frequency with which this is necessary should be expressed, and the means should be detailed.

e. Pressure area care: What type of care should be given in relation to the patient's skin type, level of hydration, nutritional status, mobility and ability to maintain certain positions? Are any aids necessary, such as ripple mattresses, sheepskins, bootees, and so on? If so, how often are these to be changed and laundered?

f. Bladder care and urinary output: Is this likely to be affected by the patient's condition? Are fluids restricted or encouraged? This has a bearing on the output, obviously. How is this to be recorded? Is the patient dehydrated or overhydrated? Is he able to go out to the toilet unaided? If not, can he walk with aid or does he need a wheelchair? Is he continent? Is he catheterised? If so, how often does he need catheter toilet? How often should the catheter be changed? Is he on diuretics? If so, how often is a urinal to be offered? Does he have polyuria? Can he pass urine supine or does he need help to stand by his bed? Does he have privacy in meeting these needs?

g. Bowel care: How often does the patient normally open his bowels? Does he normally take an aperient, and if so, which one? Does he have a condition which will influence the frequency? If so, does he need to be positioned near the toilets? Is he allowed to get up to the toilet unaided? Is he permitted to go to the toilet at night, or is a bedpan or commode necessary? Does frequency of bowel action lead to his having excoriated anal skin? If so, what medications are necessary? Are his bowel actions very offensive in smell? If so, is a deodorant spray necessary? If he tends to be constipated, perhaps through chronic illness, can this be relieved by a high fibre diet? Could he tolerate this?

h. Food and fluids needs and preferences: These may have been covered in the doctor's orders, but if not does he have any other dietary needs, perhaps dictated by culture or religion? What size appetite does he have? If appetite is poor, how is this to be remedied? How frequent is his need for food? Is he edentulous? Does he have any marked preferences and dislikes?

i. Relief of pain and discomfort: Does he have a high or low threshold for pain? Is he used to taking analgesics prior to admission? Does he have any painful conditions, e.g. piles, arthritis, etc., which are not the reason for his admission but which might nevertheless need care and attention?

j. Sight and hearing: Are these abilities restricted in any way? If he is partially sighted, does his bed need to be moved to enable him to watch television? Does he need spectacles? Can he read the menu or consent form, for example? Can he hear what is said to him?

3. Specific needs related to his hospitalisation:

a. Is ward noise a problem to him? Is he unable to sleep due to this? Should his bed be moved away from the nurse's station (for example), or away from the entrance to the dirty utility room?

b. Are the neighbouring patients congenial to him? If he is young, is he placed near the elderly or dying?

c. Is the furniture appropriate for him? If he is arthritic or paralysed, is his bed or chair too high? If very tall, is the bed too short? If he has a back lesion, is the bed too soft? If he has a painful condition, is his bed in a position where it might be bumped or jolted? If he is on a Stryker frame, is he in a position where he can see what is going on? Does he have the necessary aids? Is he in a draught, or too close to a radiator? If paralysed or receiving an intravenous infusion, is his locker on the correct side? Is his property well safeguarded? Can he easily reach his bell, or if aphasic his pad and pencil?

4. Needs for safety:

a. If he is confused or disorientated or paralysed, does he need cotsides? Is the floor sufficiently non-slip if he has problems in walking? If he uses a stick, is the ferrule worn or slippery? Does he need a stool to enable him to get in and out of bed? If he is allowed to smoke, is he safe? Has he an ashtray? Is there oxygen in use anywhere on the ward? Does he need help in using potentially dangerous equipment, such as a razor? Does he have areas of impaired sensation, which prevent him from appreciating danger? Is he likely to burn himself, or scald himself on hot drinks?

5. The need to prevent complications:
   a. What precautions are necessary in order to prevent, for example, contractures, bed sores, deep vein thromboses, wound infections, drug reactions, hypostatic pneumonia, urinary tract infections, constipation, malfunction of intravenous apparatus or drainage apparatus? How might complications be recognised?
6. The need to work with others in the caring team:
   a. Does the patient need physiotherapy? How often is the administration of such treatment necessary? What form does it take? Who is to carry on this care in the evenings and weekends?
   b. Is occupational therapy necessary? What form is it to take? Is help necessary or even desirable?
   c. Is speech therapy necessary? If so, how can the nurses best carry on the work in the absence of the therapist?
7. The need to involve the patient:
   a. What information needs to be given to the patient or his relatives? What does *he* want to know? (these two aspects may differ in content). Here one needs to take into account the patient's age, temperament and intellect. Who is to give this information? Where is the information given to be recorded? Does he need general health education? Does he need disease- or treatment-related teaching? If so, at what level? Does he need to be instructed in the use of special equipment or prostheses? How often does he need reinforcement? How much help does he need in order to accept limitations? By whom? How long is it estimated that this will take?
8. Psychological needs:
   a. All patients need privacy, but does he have particular needs, for example in the wearing of prostheses? Is he shy or embarrassed by intimate contact? Does he need solitude or companionship? Does he need protection from too many visitors who stay too long? Does he need an opportunity for private discussion with his family? How does he react to his disease? What defence mechanisms does he use: denial, projection, repression, sublimation? Does he appear overly anxious or fearful? How much encouragement does he need? Is he easily depressed by setbacks? Is he disproportionately cheerful? Is he lonely? What makes him likeable or less popular than other patients? What are his overt and covert needs in this area?

9. Spiritual needs:
   a. Does he have a need to see the hospital chaplain or a prac-
      titioner of the appropriate faith? Is there likely to be a need
      dictated by his condition, any intervention or his prognosis?
      Are there any associated dietary or procedural needs?
10. Needs on discharge:
   a. What does he need in order to carry on life outside hos-
      pital? For instance, does he need drugs, special equipment,
      contact with specialised agencies, advice? In which areas
      will he need advice – dietary needs, level of day-to-day
      activity, mobility, exercise, sexual activity? How soon
      should he see his own GP? How soon should he have
      hospital follow-up?

Planning care does not have to be the lengthy, and somewhat
academic, exercise that it seems at first sight. The use of a nursing
model based on nursing theory provides an intellectual framework
for the nurse in the provision of care, so that she can prescribe care
specific to the individual and so that, when necessary, other nurses
can take over the patient's care and maintain the standards set.
With frequent use, this approach to planning care becomes inter-
nalised and second nature. Some twenty or thirty years ago, *treatment* was built very much around a medical model; now, we can
see *care* being built very much around a nursing model.

This approach to care appears to be more time-consuming, but
if it goes some way towards meeting the needs of the individual
patient with a concurrent rise in the standards of care given, then
an appreciable rise in job satisfaction for the nurse will follow.

Intervention

Having planned care and set objectives, only then is one in a
position to intervene and implement care. Too frequently in the
past, scant attention was paid to the preceding stages of the
process, and intervention followed almost directly on admission of
the patient. Implementation implies the actual delivery of care, and
it is obvious that this is of little value unless it is appropriate.

From what has gone before, it is evident that in nursing today
we are endeavouring to consider the total patient: to look at the
person as a whole, and thus to make care a comprehensive bio-
psycho-social exercise.

This is, of course, an exercise most relevant to the type of ward organisation where patient allocation exists rather than task allocation. For instance, where the latter style of nursing care prevails, it is by no means easy to give full and all-embracing care to a patient who is looked after by a series of nurses, each of whom is concerned with a different aspect of his functioning. If one nurse takes the patient's temperature, another his blood pressure, another performs his wound dressing, and yet another his catheter toilet, then he is not in a position to build up a continuing, rewarding relationship with any one of them, nor they with him. It is, therefore, encouraging that attempts have been made recently in most hospitals within the United Kingdom to move from a task allocation system to total patient care by individuals for individuals.

Each action and each skill performed by the nurse at this stage must be individualised. Removing a T-tube from Mrx X is different in many respects from performing the same act for Mrs Y. Mrs X may have a lower pain threshold; may have arthritis, and therefore be unable to move to the correct position with ease; may be excessively anxious; or may be hard of hearing. The skill required in each case, therefore, is totally different, and is entirely related to the patient's own particular needs.

This stage of individualised nursing care requires of the nurse skills different again from either of the two preceding stages – and essentially they are the skills of a good manager.

Implementation involves management decisions as to who should deliver care, and delegation of care to members of the nursing care team as appropriate. It therefore demands of the team leader skill in assessing the strengths and limitations of each member of her staff, and skills in determining the level of expertise required to deliver care to individual patients.

Evaluation

Evaluation is testing the outcome of the actions against the previously anticipated outcomes. This is the final stage of individualised care planning. Having said that, though, one should not be misled into the belief that it occurs only at the end of the patient's care phase. Evaluation must occur concurrently with planning and implementation. It is the crucial tool for updating the care plan and ensuring that the care delivered is both necessary and appropriate. The frequency of evaluation depends on the patient's condition.

At this stage, what is it that we are evaluating? We should be considering the patient's progress in terms of his response to treatment, both medical and nursing; the alteration, if any, in his diagnoses; his response to hospitalisation; his response to the care as planned; the quality and standard of the care given; and finally, the nurse should be evaluating herself in the delivery of that care.

It involves going back once more to the stages of assessment of needs and planning of care. One needs to look again at the patient's needs to see if they have been met by executing the care specified at the planning stage; and thus one needs to assess the degree to which one's objectives have been met.

American literature gives several ideas for fairly sophisticated methods of carrying out evaluation (Phaneuf, 1969), for example, the nursing audit. This is defined as the formal and systematic written appraisal of the quality of nursing service indicated in the care records of discharged patients. Systems analysis may be used, or more simply the patient interview and observation by the nurse who checks continuously the care delivered against the care plan.

Evaluation allows the nurse to assess her own performance, not only in delivering care but also in assessing the patient's needs. The patient's view should not be forgotten at this stage, as he is often best placed to assess the effectiveness of his needs' satisfaction.

In evaluating care, the nurse should go back to the stage where the nursing objectives were set. These should:

a. identify measurable, observable behaviour that can be accepted as evidence of the desired outcome.
b. define the important conditions under which the behaviour is to occur.
c. define the criteria of acceptable performance, bearing in mind the limitations of the individual.

The adequacy of the objectives, therefore, influences not only the quality of care but also the ease with which that care can be evaluated.

The skills required at this stage are thus those of assessing objectives and measuring the degree to which these have been met, skills in replanning care to meet re-assessed needs, and, finally, skills of objective self-assessment in determining how well the nurse has exercised her clinical skills. The whole can be seen to require considerable clinical judgment which comes with skilled teaching and experience.

These stages of assessment, planning, intervention and evaluation characteristic of the delivery of individual patient care can be seen as tools: tools that enable us to give the kind of care which defines the best professional nursing, and which enable us to unlock the door to the patient's problems, to discuss and to attend to his needs.

With the increasing sophistication of treatment available today in both the medical and nursing spheres, there emerges an even greater battery of needs on the part of the patient.

It was Florence Nightingale who said that 'the very elements of nursing are all but unknown'. We may still not have reached a definition of nursing that satisfies all criteria; nevertheless, if we have gone some way towards meeting patients' needs in a comprehensive and organised way, then we have come nearer to knowing more about the very elements of nursing.

REFERENCES

Abdellah, F. G. et al (1960) *Patient Centred Approaches to Nursing*. New York: Macmillan.
Boore, J. (1978) *A prescription for recovery*. London: Royal College of Nursing.
Hay, Stella, I. & Anderson, Helen, C. (1963) Are nurses meeting patients' needs? *American Journal of Nursing*, **63**, 96–99.
Hayward, J. (1975) *Information – A prescription against pain*. London: Royal College of Nursing.
Henderson, V. (1958) *Basic Principles of Nursing Care*. London: International Council of Nurses.
Henderson, V. (1966) *The Nature of Nursing*. London: Collier Macmillan.
Maslow, A. H. (1970) *Motivation and Personality*, 2nd edition. New York and London: Harper and Row.
Nightingale, Florence (1859) *Notes on Nursing*. 1970 edition, pp. 13, 59. London: Duckworth.
Norton, D. (1975) *An Investigation of Geriatric Nursing Problems in Hospital*. Edinburgh: Churchill Livingstone.
Phaneuf, Maria, C. (1966) The nursing audit for evaluation of patient care. *Nursing Outlook*, **14**, (6), 51–54.
Riehl, J. & Roy, C. 1980 *Conceptual Models for Nursing Practice* New York: Appleton-Century-Crofts.
Wolff, H. & Erickson, R. (1977) The assessment man. *Nursing Outlook*, **25**, (2).

FURTHER READING

Auld & Birum (1973) *The Challenge of Nursing*. Saint Louis: C.V. Mosby Company.
Bailey, J. & Claus, K. (1975) *Decision Making in Nursing – Tools for Change*. Saint Louis: C.V. Mosby Company.
Brown, Esther Lucille (1970) *Nursing Reconsidered: A Study of Change*. Philadelphia: Lippincott.

Gebbie, K. M. & Lavin, M. A. (1975) *Classification of Nursing Diagnoses*. Saint Louis: C.V. Mosby Company.

Gooding, Marion Brown (1972) *Techniques for Utilising Nursing Principles*. Saint Louis: C.V. Mosby Company.

Hollingworth, S. (1985) *Preparation for Change*. London: Royal College of Nursing.

Hunt, J. & Marks-Maran, D. (1980) *Nursing Care Plans – the Nursing Process at Work*. London: H.M. & M. Publishers.

LeLean, Sylvia (1973) *Ready for Report, Nurse?* Royal College of Nursing Research Project.

McFarlane, J. (Baroness) & Casteldine, G. (1982) *A Guide to the Practice of Nursing – Using the Nursing Process*. Saint Louis: C.V. Mosby Company.

Marriner, Ann (1975) *The Nursing Process: A Scientific Approach to Nursing Care*. Saint Louis: C.V. Mosby Company.

Nightingale, Florence (1859) *Notes on Nursing*. Facsimile edition 1970. London: Duckworth.

Orem, D. (1980) *Nursing, Concepts of Practice*. New York: McGraw Hill.

Roper, N., Logan, W. & Tierney, A. (1985) *Learning to Use the Process of Nursing* 2nd edn. Edinburgh: Churchill Livingstone.

Stockwell, Felicity (1972) *The Unpopular Patient*. Royal College of Nursing Research Project.

Vitale, Schultz & Nugent (1974) *A Problem Solving Approach to Nursing Care Plans: A Program*. Saint Louis: C.V. Mosby Company.

2

The role of the teacher in the clinical field

The following are two letters from student nurses. The reader is left to draw her own conclusions after reading them.

Dear Sandra,
I arrived on the ward this morning, late as usual. Since I've been here I don't sleep very well, and last night I forgot to set my alarm. The reception I got on the ward was very cool, even though I tried to apologise for my lateness. There had been no report from the night staff, so I hadn't missed much. The first catastrophe was when a lady who was due for an operation this morning had been given a cup of tea by one of the very junior pupil nurses. The latter got a real rocket, but (as she said) there was no sign over the bed, and nobody had said the patient was to have nil by mouth. The nurse whispered quietly to me that she didn't really understand what the danger was. I tried to explain it to her, but I was called away to help give an injection. I'd not done many of these, and hoped the staff nurse would let me try – but she said everyone was too busy, and that she could do it quicker. I trailed along behind her, quite sure I shouldn't have signed the Controlled Drugs Book until the injection had been given – but she said very icily that she knew what she was doing, and insisted that I did what I was told. After that, I didn't dare say that I couldn't read the name on the ampoule, so I've no idea really what we gave the patient. The lady seemed very frightened and anxious when she had had the injection, even though the staff nurse had explained its effect. I did feel a smile might have helped. Still, I'm only small fry, and have a lot to learn. I suppose people in hospital expect 'cool efficiency', and not a lot of chatter about nothing.
  After this injection, the staff nurse left me and joined one of her colleagues. They were having a good old chat whilst bathing a very lively patient so I thought I should find another nurse to help me bath Mr Smith. He's very ill and has been with us some time. I'm

not sure exactly how long, as I've never heard all his case history, and some of the notes are very difficult to read. He's got See A; I think that's what the abbreviation is, but I'm not sure where. Anyway, I feel I know him quite well now, as most mornings I seem to give him his wash. It was rather a shock when I first saw his shrunken little body, but Sister said we've got to try to make him eat and drink as much as possible. He has a high protein diet, and unfortunately one of his meals was eaten by someone else the other day. I went to look for it when I realised nobody was feeding him, and found Mr Ponsonby was half-way through it. When I told the senior student, she didn't seem to know quite what to do as we were so busy. But I found some eggs and mixed those up in some milk. Mr Smith seemed to enjoy that.

Anyway, it looked as if there was just the pupil nurse free, and she seemed very willing to give me a hand as she hadn't really been given anything to do. Together we managed to wash most of Mr Smith, but had difficulty in moving him as he seemed in so much pain. We did our best, but wished that someone more senior had come just to make sure we were doing things correctly. I didn't realise until later that day that although the pupil nurse had been on the ward longer than me she couldn't really tell me any more about Mr Smith than I knew already.

By lunch-time most of the work seemed to be finished. I felt that I had worked really hard and had done the best I could for the patients, but somehow it was dfficult to finish one job properly before something else needed doing. Someone was constantly telling me 'it's nearly twelve o'clock'. At least the patients seemed grateful and their 'thank you's' made up for all the criticism, especially when you feel you could do it better with a little more help. By lunch-time I was feeling very tired and dejected. I expect that was why I forgot of fill in the fluid charts. I got such a telling off for that as soon as I set foot in the ward after lunch. I remember that they said it was important in the school, but some days no one seems to notice whether they are filled up or not!

The ward seemed fairly quiet for a couple of hours, so we were allowed to look at the patients' notes. The writing is so difficult to read sometimes, and all the abbreviations are like a foreign language. If only somebody could have explained them a bit I might not have been caught gazing out of the window. Oh dear, they must think I'm stupid or uninterested, or both. I worry about it when I'm off duty but don't feel that I can talk to the ward staff as they seem to have problems of their own. It is now way past my bed-time and I must put out the light. No wonder I oversleep so easily.

Hope things are more cheerful with you.

Love, Alison.

Dear Alison,

I arrived on the ward late this morning – my alarm clock just did not go off. Anyway, the ward sister accepted my explanation and sent me to early coffee when she discovered I had not had breakfast. She always seems concerned about her nurses, and I must say I felt better after eating something. After we had dealt with the patients' breakfasts, we had then a report on the patients we would be looking after for the day. We used the care plans in the kardex to check on current problems. The staff nurse I worked with said we have to take special note of those patients who can have nothing by mouth before operation. It makes you really careful when you know what could happen to a patient who was given something by accident.

One lady was going to the theatre this morning and as we had been told yesterday, she was very anxious. We were all asked to try to help her by being kind, understanding and giving repeated explanations about what was happening to her. I've had to look after little Mr Brown quite a lot during my first week. He is very ill, and has a cancer in his stomach. The nurses all seem very fond of him, even when he gets irritable and rude. Sister helped me when I first bathed him in bed, and showed me the way to lift him so that it wouldn't hurt. It was so satisfying when we had finished. He was clean, comfortable and warm. We'd also shared a few laughs with him about this and that, which seemed to lift his spirits somewhat.

This morning, though, a staff nurse helped me and explained that we had to pass a Ryle's tube because Mr Brown was too weak to eat. She helped me to assemble the equipment in the treatment room, and explained how the procedure was to be carried out. It seemed so clear I felt that I could do it myself – which is just what happened. She suggested that I should pass the tube under her supervision. Well, I was nervous, but she put me at my ease and everything went well. We gave Mr Brown his tube feed and I was reminded to write the amount given accurately on his fluid chart. Sister asked me about the procedure later, making sure I knew why it had been necessary. She didn't seem to mind my lack of 'technical jargon', but made sure I had added some more long words to the ever-increasing list in the back of my notebook. She also showed me briefly one of the ward textbooks, in which I would find a very useful chapter on the nursing care required for very sick patients.

When all the care required by our patients was completed, and all the patients' observation charts were up to date, we went to lunch. Just as well, as I was starving!

The afternoon was a little less hectic, and there was time for the clinical teacher to give two of us a tutorial. As we had several diabetic patients on the ward, we talked about the two different types (diabetes mellitus and diabetes insipidus). It was very interesting, and we used the patients' nursing assessment sheet, notes and kardex as a basis for working out their problems, actual and potential. From here we were able to discuss the care plan which would be most appropriate for the patient and the methods by which the care would be carried out and evaluated. In particular we talked about insulin. The penny really dropped about drawing up insulin. I feel so pleased to think that this procedure may no longer be quite so frightening – even though you know another senior nurse is always present. At the end of the session, the clinical teacher gave us some tutorial notes on a little card with a diagram of the pancreas and a book reference on the back. Sometimes she brings us books from the library, which saves us quite a walk. If she makes an effort like that, the least I can do is to read the relevant chapter for her.

Everyone on the ward is so enthusiastic about nursing and it's difficult not to 'catch' this feeling. Even when the ward is really busy, I still feel that I am an important member of the team. I suppose it's because they explain things to me, and show me how to practise nursing skills which I've not seen before. I never feel left out. My written list of ward learning objectives helps me to understand more about the patients' total care. The ward teaching sessions are linked to these objectives. Each week a list is put up and everyone is encouraged to be responsible for teaching – even I have to contribute in a tutorial next week!

Anyway, I must just read this chapter before I put the light out – no doubt Sister will want to know whether I have any queries about it tomorrow. With any luck I may be able to give some insulin injections with her some time. She is so kind to the patients and if I can master just some of her skills I will be very pleased.

Still, I must get to my books – hope all is as happy on your new ward.
Much love, in haste, Sandra.

What is the role of the teacher in the clinical field?

'Roles are families of expectancies'. (Kretch, Crutchfield & Ballachy 1962.)

The role of any teacher is to help people to learn. This is especially true when considering a teacher who is working in the clinical field of nursing. Teachers, in this context, include all members of staff from senior nursing officers to junior pupil and student nurses. Each member should be concerned with teaching in one way or another. It is her responsibility to help, guide and support those people, patients, hospital personnel, relatives etc., with whom she comes into contact. Often this function is carried out quite adequately without the 'teacher' being aware of exactly what she is doing. Some members of the hospital team, however, are more familiar with teaching methods having gained formal qualifications on various courses.

The role of the teacher in the clinical field has a direct effect on patient care. How are nursing skills being carried out? Does the learner perform safely, kindly and with confidence? Is she aware of the reason why a particular nursing skill is carried out in a certain manner? Bad habits are picked up so quickly, and without the clinical judgement and help which the ward staff give to their learners, a patient's life or certainly his well-being could be at risk.

The person who is ill must remain at the centre of each individual's awareness. It is this fact which prompts an experienced clinical teacher, staff nurse or ward sister to watch a learner at work, and try to ensure that her nursing skills are developing correctly. Left to her own devices, an uncertain junior nurse will usually attempt a procedure to the best of her ability; but 'trial and error' learning (as we shall see) can have a dangerous and sometimes painful effect on the patient.

Whilst working in the clinical area the learner needs to feel secure in herself and also secure with those around her. Although we aim to eliminate mistakes when sick people are being cared for, unfortunately they do, and will continue occasionally to occur. Sometimes the reason can be traced back to insufficient instruction and explanation, or maybe the nurse was too frightened to ask for the help she clearly needed. A mistake could on the other hand have stemmed from a nursing report or care plan heavily laden with abbreviations. One example is that of a young nurse who interpreted an 'I.V. infusion' as being a distillation of ivy, which grows on so many hospital walls! Oversights like these do lead learners to experience intense anxiety on the ward, especially if they do not consider that the ward atmosphere lends itself to asking questions. Time is everyone's enemy, but perhaps as teachers we hide behind this too much and indeed, now that many ward duties have been designated 'non-nursing' duties, we should have more time to spare. Although the levels of staffing invariably fluctuate from time to time, a high standard of patient care is dependent on a sound understanding of what needs to be done, and why it is important to do it, rather than on a high staff-patient ratio *per se*.

A sterile dressing is a good example of this point, as the cost of poor technique to both patient and the National Health Service is great. All members of the teaching team in the clinical field must set an example, by allowing learners to see the procedures being carried out: not only swiftly and skilfully, but safely.

Each member of the ward teaching team carries a wide range of responsibilities. The senior nurse concerned with the smooth running of her unit is invaluable as a teacher, as she has many years of clinical experience behind her. It is often of great value to ask her to speak to groups of learners in the school of nursing.

This can be particularly helpful to the students before the start of their clinical experience on her particular unit.

The senior nurses might also be able to contribute to the unit tutorial team, taking a turn at holding teaching sessions on a particular aspect of the work on the unit.

The ward sister is a vital member of the teaching team. It is she who maintains and evaluates the standard of nursing care on her ward. Her first responsibility is of course to her patients, and because she possesses the skills to look after them, her example should stand out very clearly for all the learners to follow. She provides a role model. This has been well documented in recent research reports: 'The Ward Sister, Key to Nursing' (Pembrey 1980) highlights the importance of the ward sister's (or charge nurse's) managerial role in relation to the delivery of patient care; Margaret Ogier's 'The Ideal Sister' (Ogier 1981) is a study of leadership style and verbal interaction between ward sisters and nurse learners; while Helen Orton's study 'Ward learning climate' (Orton 1981) investigated a similar topic.

These and other studies emphasise the importance of the ward sister's contribution to the education and training of learners. They also describe situations in which learners are not encouraged to learn.

Reports of this kind should enable sisters and charge nurses to look constructively at their own teaching methods and also at their own wards as learning environments.

NB Teaching is not just talking. There is so much that is best learned by 'doing'.

Staff nurses, under the guidance perhaps of their ward sisters and clinical teacher, are often very good and enthusiastic nurses. It is always heartening to see their teaching skills blossom and with help they can develop their talents for being able to explain matters clearly and concisely to both patients and students alike.

Clinical teachers at present have the advantage of having spent some time on a formal course of preparation. Much of the examinable course material on the six-month full-time course is concerned with the altered physiology of the body in disease and how this may best be taught. Psychology, clinical teaching methods and practice plus other interesting topics make up the rest of the course.

From a survey of clinical teachers carried out by the Royal College of Nursing in 1975, it appeared they were very appreciative of the course, but were discontented with the extent to which they were able to use their hard-earned knowledge for the benefit of the learners.

Many felt that no one was really aware of what their course entailed. 'Failed tutors' was a comment several made, referring to how they felt their colleagues saw them; others thought that there was little opportunity to use their knowledge for ward tutorials. Their work is mainly to help learners achieve and maintain high standards of nursing care, but many clinical teachers (as the survey shows) feel like extra pairs of hands on the ward.

Generally speaking, clinical teachers work very hard, enjoying uninterrupted periods of total nursing care with their learners; but they also need time to discuss with learners the patients, their diagnoses, problems and care plans, and to consolidate the students' learning.

The present lack of a career structure for clinical teachers was also seen by some as a drawback. This seems a great pity and maybe the answer might lie in the long-awaited role of the clinical nurse specialist. Could this position provide a career development for experienced clinical teachers? This could be an answer for the clinical teacher who wrote 'after two and a half years of clinical teaching, I've been able to achieve absolutely nothing. Any ideas I do have are promised a hearing which never materialises.'

Many comments in the survey previously referred to were in a similar vein, and these indicate that the breadth of the role of the clinical teacher (in which the teaching of practical skills and nursing theory is combined) is not being fully appreciated.

Although the opportunities for teaching should make the job particularly satisfying, they can be severely limited by lack of guidance, direction and support at local level. There are many skills that a clinical teacher can bring to the ward, i.e. building good relationships, counselling, supporting, advising, etc., and she should be given every opportunity to exercise and develop all of these.

The 'one to one' situation in which the clinical teacher works should enable her to get to know the learners thoroughly and to help them with their individual problems. Sometimes, these are not all directly related to work.

Tutors still carry a heavy responsibility for the learning which takes place in the classroom. They must convey to all learners the basic concepts of nursing. If there are insufficient tutors it can be very difficult for them to visit the wards and to work with the learners themselves. To many tutors this is a great loss, as often the best possible place to demonstrate nursing skills is at the bedside. Here the presence of the patient is a very real advantage.

The link between theory and practice, the school of nursing and the ward, can therefore become very fragile. In some clinical areas, tutors are able to concentrate their knowledge and skills on particular specialities, and to forge a strong link between theory and practice. Some tutors no doubt would not support this idea, but most would agree that there are difficulties in having to be 'a jack of all trades', i.e. keeping up with all the nursing specialities.

This is not to say the tutor is not capable of teaching any given subject, but rather that complete expertise in every area of nursing is expecting a lot.

Perhaps the only answer to the problem is to abandon the two separate roles of the clinical teacher and the tutor and create one: that of a nurse teacher. Within this role, the two elements of classroom and bedside teaching could be merged. This might enable the clinical teacher to use her knowledge in the classroom and enable the 'tutor' to get her sleeves rolled up, so that she can teach the learners nursing skills on the ward.

The roles of all members of the clinical teaching team could be summarised as follows.

The teacher must:

1. be a skilled, experienced nurse, concerned to maintain and improve standards of patient care.
2. be concerned to help learners develop their potential as nurses.
3. demonstrate expertise in caring for patients.
4. show skills in teaching individuals and small groups.
5. create a favourable climate for learning.
6. be alert to learning opportunities in the ward.

How can the role be achieved?

'Force of habit – one of the four grounds of human ignorance, one of the four great obstacles to learning.' (Friar Roger Bacon. 1259.)

Having tried to establish what is involved in the role of the teacher in the clinical field, we must consider some of the ways in which it can be achieved.

One influential psychologist, Abraham Maslow (Maslow, 1970) proposed a 'hierarchy of needs', which can give the teacher a firm basis on which to develop the learning skills needed by learners. These needs seem especially relevant in the clinical field.

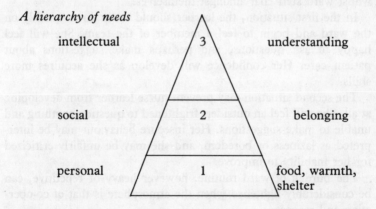

A hierarchy of needs

intellectual	3	understanding
social	2	belonging
personal	1	food, warmth, shelter

Maslow suggests that effective learning cannot take place unless the hierarchy of needs has been met. Level one is based on personal physiological needs such as food, warmth, safety and comfort. Following these considerations, level two includes the importance of self-esteem and the need to belong to a group (affiliation). Level three, dependent for its fulfilment upon the other two levels, shows a need for intellectual challenge and the ability to understand relevant material.

We can apply these ideas to nurses in training.

Level one suggests a nurse on her first ward. A young nurse nearly fainted on her first morning, as she had felt too nervous to eat breakfast. After her coffee break, she felt much better and was grateful to the ward sister who had noticed her pale face and trembling hands.

Another example of this would be the practical plea made to all new nurses: 'please choose a sensible pair of shoes'. Nobody will learn anything if her feet are killing her! So many common sense precautions need to be taken to satisfy 'needs' in level one.

Level two suggests that all learners need to feel welcome, especially if they are feeling apprehensive. For learning to take place, a relationship must be established in which the learner feels secure. We cannot exactly offer champagne and oysters, but a warm smile can mean everything to a learner during those first few days.

Sometimes ward staff can pick out very quickly those learners who need extra encouragement to do well. Unfortunately sometimes the learners are left to get on with things in total isolation whilst ward staff chat amongst themselves.

In the first situation, the learner should settle down quickly on the ward and begin to feel a member of the team. She will feel happy to ask questions, and perhaps make suggestions about patient care. Her confidence will develop as she acquires more skills.

The second situation may prevent nurse learner from developing at all. She will feel an outsider, frightened to question anything and unable to make suggestions. Her insecure behaviour may be interpreted as laziness or boredom, and she may be unfairly criticized for her inability to improve.

The burden of ward routine, however heavy or repetitive, can be considerably lightened when the atmosphere is that of co-operation and respect.

Level three of the hierarchy highlights the intellectual needs of a learner. These needs require careful assessment by the ward staff, and they are in the unique position of knowing the learning opportunities which the ward can offer.

Much of the learning will be concerned with manual dexterity, but the intellectual component of this is often considerable. Every effort must be made to ensure that the learner is able to be successful when carrying out nursing skills. It is unfair to subject her to a situation in which she may fail through lack of support.

The nursing report provides a good opportunity to assess the learner's knowledge. So often in the past, this was a one way session with the qualified ward staff talking all the time and the learners remaining silent. Increasingly nowadays, however, it provides a forum for all the nurses caring for a group of patients to discuss individually and in concert the rationale for the nursing care prescribed.

Clinical teachers and tutors frequently request formal written work from the learner. This should always be set at the right level, stimulating the learner's need to understand and to solve problems of patient care. The results of this work should be returned as soon as possible, so that the learner's interest will not wane.

Many learners are concerned about the lack of ward teaching. This was shown in John Birch's study, *To nurse or not to nurse* (1975).

It must be said that many students and pupils do not recognise any activity which they see, whilst standing on their feet, as teaching. Their perception of teaching relates only to the classroom where they are seated and engaged in listening. Learning by example has potential which the learners frequently need to have pointed out to them. A ward demonstration of good nursing care is a valuable piece of teaching.

In order to compliment the teacher's appreciation of Maslow's hierarchy of needs, it is also important that the student or pupil nurse should develop a more discerning judgement of different types of teaching, and attempt to benefit from all of them.

To develop teaching skills further, it is useful to mention one or two theories of learning which have been well documented.

J. B. Watson outlined a process of 'trial and error' learning. He put forward the thesis that, in spite of initial and inevitable mistakes being made, a person could eventually solve problems provided that rewards were offered every time a correct attempt was made.

Applying this to the clinical field has obvious limitations, and we must be careful to protect the patients from the effects of too much 'trial and error'. This learning theory is best used in the classroom and practical room where learners can recognise and benefit from their mistakes before involving their patients. Manual dexterity is not always inborn, and often nurse learners need to practise before they feel happy to perform the real thing.

Ivan Pavlov is best remembered for his work on classical conditioning. Whilst carrying out psychological studies on dogs, he noted that they salivated immediately before they were fed. This he called an 'unconditioned response'. He extended this idea by repeatedly ringing a bell each time the dogs were fed. Following this experiment, he was able to demonstrate that the dogs would salivate to the sound of a ringing bell. This he called a 'conditioned response'.

In diagrammatic form, the process could be represented as follows:

Stimulus	Organism	Response	
Food	Organism	Salivation	Unconditioned response
Bell	Organism	Salivation	Conditioned response

This psychological theory can be related to human activity, largely in terms of the body's automatic responses. In the learning environment, its value is limited as rather a simplistic idea:

Stimulus	Organism	Response	
Teacher is pleasant	Organism	Happy in class	Unconditioned response
Work	Organism	Happy to work	Conditioned response

This theory is heavily dependent on reflex action and emotional activity, and cannot in isolation be used in the clinical field.

B.F. Skinner's contribution to the theories of learning have been widely documented. Like Pavlov, his interest is in conditioning, but his main work has been on 'operant conditioning'. This idea relates to a person's behaviour being shaped rather than simply conditioned. A task performed well will receive positive reinforcement and is more likely to be repeated. A task which is poorly carried out will receive negative reinforcement and the behaviour is therefore likely to be extinguished.

Applied to the teaching of learners in the clinical field, this theory means that the teacher might constantly be trying to shape the learners' behaviour towards the right methods and to extinguish slapdash delivery of care.

Force of habit, as said earlier, is one of the great obstacles to learning, and all teachers must ensure that bad habits are not allowed to develop.

This theory also allows for the learner carrying out nursing care in small steps, and receiving feedback on her success at each stage. Knowledge of results is important, especially when teaching the intricate skills of nursing.

Teaching in small steps contrasts quite well with learning in large chunks. Psychologists such as Koffka, Kohler and Wertheimer were concerned with the school of Gestalt psychology, that is, seeing things as a whole, the whole being greater than the sum of the constituent parts.

Gestalt theory relies heavily on the use of the learner's past experience, her correct perception of the present situation, and her movement from 'known' to 'unknown'.

In the ward this means that the teacher needs to know what the learner has experienced before. She must also ensure that what she is seeing, hearing or saying is clear and accurate.

Whilst watching a clinical procedure, the learner will gain little if she is watching from too far away or from the wrong side of the bed. She also needs to be able to ask questions to make sure that her interpretation of what has been seen is correct. In this way, the learner will be able to fit new information into the pattern of that which she already possesses. This process can often result in a motivating 'penny-dropping' moment, when suddenly a perceptual pattern is completed. 'Oh, *that's* why it needs to be done like that', or '*now* I realise what the equipment is there for'. This experience in itself provides positive reinforcement to the learner.

Events like this are very satisfying to a teacher, and make up for some of the occasions when the drop of a penny seems a life-time away. The contribution of taxonomies (classifications) of educational objectives written by Bloom, Krathwohl, Simpson and others (Pring, 1971) has also had an enormous influence on theories of ward teaching. These taxonomies have enabled learning opportunities to be classified into cognitive, affective and psychomotor domains. The domains have provided a structure for the aims and objectives which the learner is to achieve.

Although aims and objectives provide useful tools for organising learning material, it should be remembered that they point only to one way in which this can be achieved. Other curriculum models, such as the process model, can be used (Stenhouse 1971). In this model, although general aims are used, the process of learning is different in that it allows the teacher to be more neutral and permits the learner to become more constructively critical about what she is doing.

Using objectives which dictate expected outcomes too precisely can become mechanistic. There must be room for imaginative and creative learning. The objectives need to be written by the ward staff together with the tutorial staff to ensure that they are realistic and appropriate.

With some knowledge of these theories of learning, we could fit them into a learning process.

Borrowed directly from the nursing process, the steps would be:

1. Assess (the learning needs)
2. Plan (the learning plan)
3. Carry out (the learning plan)
4. Evaluate (the learning plan)

Assessing an individual's learning needs involves all the teaching team in deciding what it is that we expect the learner to be able to do on the ward. This involves working out general aims, and more particularly, learning objectives. An example of the latter might be 'The learner will carry out unaided an aseptic technique on a simple undrained wound, with optimum safety within a specified time limit.'

The principle here is that by setting objectives in behavioural terms (i.e. what the learner should be capable of doing), her activity becomes observable and measurable. Each task expected of the learner should be carefully worked out in advance of her arrival, stating clearly the criteria by which each objective should be achieved.

The needs of the learner should also be considered, requiring a knowledge of the past experience which she will be bringing with her to the ward. She may be very junior, or a nurse approaching her final examinations. The generality of aims and objectives must not obscure the individuality of each learner.

Careful assessment of potential learning opportunities can be augmented by a learning plan. This might take the form of an individual sheet on which the learner finds her name against a selection of patients for whom she must prepare a care plan (this would also relate to the ward learning objectives).

It is her responsibility (with the guidance and supervision of the ward and tutorial staff) to present her work and to demonstrate her ability to implement and evaluate total patient care. The learner then has an individual record of her professional skills, which should be discussed with her regularly.

Evaluation is always time consuming, but necessary in order to maintain and monitor the process. Did the learner achieve what was expected of her? If not, why not? Were the learning objectives appropriate, observable and measurable? Not all nursing activities can be measured – for example, those concerned with human relationships. These may need to be evaluated by different methods.

A study of learning theories, and a consideration of learning as a process, can form a basis for most clinical teaching, which should allow an active response to be made by the learner rather than a passive assimilation of activities going on round her.

Knowledge of this kind could benefit all members of the teaching team. It would give added insight to those who have a natural gift for communicating with and relating to students; and perhaps more confidence to those who find the prospect of teaching somewhat daunting.

In-service teaching courses, however short, are a necessity. The syllabus should include:

1. An introduction to the principles of teaching
   a. The requirements for learning; interest, motivation, activity, knowledge of results.
   b. The nature of learning
      (i) Trial and error
      (ii) Conditioning
      (iii) Insight
   c. The characteristics of a skilled performance and the acquisition of skills.
   d. Individual and group activities
   e. Individual differences in intelligence, age, attitude, language, culture.
2. Methods of teaching
   a. curriculum design
   b. preparation, content, visual aids
   c. teaching method, demonstration, project work, tutorials, role play, independent study
   d. assessment of learners' work.

These and other topics are included in ENB Course No 998 –

Teaching and Assessing in Clinical Practice – which is now being offered by many Schools of Nursing to nurses, midwives and health visitors who have responsibility for teaching, supervising and assessing students in the clinical setting.

Why is the role important

'The worst sin against our fellow creatures is not to hate them, but to be indifferent to them: that's the essence of inhumanity'. (*Devil's Disciple*, Bernard Shaw)

The role of any teacher is one of privilege and importance; for nurses to be good teachers is especially important. They have a dual function: the care of the sick individual and care of the learner. They should not be indifferent to either. Both the patient and the learner have needs which must be anticipated and met.

The importance of good teaching in the clinical field is that it offers a vital contribution to the maintenance and constant evaluation of standards for patient care.

REFERENCES

Birch, J. (1975) *To Nurse or not to Nurse*. London: Royal College of Nursing.
Kretch, Crutchfield & Ballachey (1962) *Individuals in Society*. New York: McGraw Hill.
Maslow, A. (1970) *Motivation and Personality*, 2nd edn. New York and London: Harper and Row.
Ogier, M. (1981) *An Ideal Sister*. London: Royal College of Nursing.
Orton, H. (1981) *Ward Learning Climate*. London: Royal College of Nursing.
Pembrey, S. (1980) *The Ward Sister, Key to Nursing*. London: Royal College of Nursing.
Pring, R. (1971) Bloom's Taxonomy, a philosophical critique. *Cambridge Journal of Education*, No. 2.
Stenhouse, L. (1975) *An Introduction to Curriculum Research and Development*. London: Heinemann.

FURTHER READING

Carr, A. J. (1977) Clinical nurse teaching. *Nursing Times*, January 27.
Child, D. (1976) *Psychology and the Teacher*. London: Holt-Blond Ltd.
Eisner, E. W. (1977) Instructional and expressive objectives. In *Curriculum Design*, ed. Golby, M. London: Croom Helm.
Greaves, F. (1980) Objectively towards curriculum improvement in nurse education. *Journal of Advanced Nursing*, 5, 591–599.
Macdonald-Ross, M. (1973) Behavioural objectives – a critical review. In *Curriculum Design*, ed. Golby, M. London: Croom Helm.

Marson, S. (1982) Ward sister, teacher or facilitator. *Journal of Advanced Nursing*, 7.

Schweer, J. & Gebbie, K. (1976) *Creative Teaching in Clinical Nursing*. Saint Louis: C.V. Mosby.

Smith, L. (1982) Models of nursing as the basis for curriculum development: some rationales and implications. *Journal of Advanced Nursing*, 7, 112–127.

3

Ward learning: opportunities and problems

Nurse education is at present undergoing great changes. But whatever happens, the ward will retain an important place in training. Whether the nurse gains clinical experience in the ward as an apprentice or as a student-observer, the main aim is still to provide the best nursing care possible for the patient.

The Committee on Nursing (1972), chaired by Professor Asa Briggs, stated that it believed nursing to be the major caring profession. It follows from this that one of the main aims of nurse training must be to produce a nurse capable of a high standard of nursing care. During the three-year course for registration, the student nurse spends four-fifths of her time on clinical work. It is, therefore, in the ward that most of her experience is gained, and here that the standard of good practice is set.

This chapter explores some of the learning opportunities provided by the ward and some of the problems that may arise. The emphasis throughout is on learning rather than teaching. Included are some suggestions for making the best use of the opportunities and for overcoming the problems.

Ward learning resources

During her training, a student is assigned to various clinical areas for periods of six to twelve weeks. In line with EEC directives, the programme now includes experience of geriatric, paediatric, obstetric, psychiatric and trauma care. The community aspect of each specialty is also covered. A learner therefore has to adjust to many different environments as well as learning about a particular specialty. Too frequent changes in clinical work could produce a fragmented training and may put stress on the learner; but the more varied her experience, the more able the nurse will be in solving problems. Properly planned, each allocation will provide a new sort of experience, and by making full use of her learning opportunities the student will gain in knowledge, ability and confidence.

The ward is the ideal place for learning, but only if its full potential is realised. This raises several important issues.

The first of these is 'What has the ward to offer the learner in practical experience?' Ward objectives are invaluable here in helping to identify the practical experience. For example, one objective may be that 'by the end of the allocation the student will be able to plan the nursing care of a patient following cholecystectomy, based on his or her problems and needs'. By formulating such objectives, ward staff are able to define precisely the general and the specific care required by the patients of their particular specialty.

Because of the specialist nature of most wards, some skills will be practised by the learner only during that one allocation. Stoma care and continuous ambulatory peritoneal dialysis are examples of this. Other aspects of care, however, are common to all patients regardless of the nature of their illness. Objectives help to guide a student's learning by specifying the range of experience available.

Another consideration when formulating ward objectives is 'who is available to help to teach the students during an allocation?' The ward sister is clearly the most important person of all. The standard of nursing care, the atmosphere and the promotion of a good learning environment all depend on her. The role of the ward sister will be discussed more fully later in the chapter.

In addition, whilst in the ward, the learner has the opportunity to work in close contact with specialists in all fields. The specialist personnel, such as a physiotherapist, a clinical nurse specialist or a social worker, can help the student to learn about all aspects of patient care. The student will also learn about the importance of teamwork in the clinical field by observing the contribution of each to total patient care.

The student nurse can also learn much from the patient and his or her family. Nursing care is individual to each patient, as the patient should not be expected to conform to a set pattern of treatment. All nurses must be ready to ask the patient's advice, and not feel resentful if their care is questioned. For example, a patient with disabling rheumatoid arthritis can teach the learner the best way to perform a procedure with the minimum of discomfort. Relatives will be helpful in providing information about the home environment, thus increasing understanding of the patient. For the student to benefit from this opportunity to learn, time and encouragement must be given for informal 'chats'. Too often, quiet spells in the ward are spent in 'weekend cleaning' and not in patient contact.

Ward objectives will help to ensure that the learner's training programme is co-ordinated. The objectives should therefore be modified according to the individual requirements of a student. This brings us to another important factor in developing the full potential of the ward learning environment: 'what does the student require from the clinical experience?' A nurse working in her first ward is going to need a very different experience from a senior student preparing for her final examination. The ward specialty, however, remains the same. The requirements of all nurses must be recognised, and met by allocating the appropriate experience. Clinical assessment for learners is a useful aid here in monitoring the progress achieved.

Ward organisation is important in ensuring that the learner's individual requirements for the development of her clinical skills are met. The emphasis must be on total patient care, whereby the learner has responsibility for particular patients. The allocation of work by tasks, although an efficient way of ensuring that work is completed, is unsatisfying for both the nurse and the patient.

The patient is in hospital for treatment of disease, and obviously care is designed to promote his or her comfort and well-being. Whilst in the ward, however, a patient is also the ideal audio-visual aid for learning (Fig. 3.1). Although this role is secondary, and must at no time be abused, the student learns through planning and providing care for individual patients.

Individual care is based on an understanding of the social, psychological and physical condition of the patient. He or she may have several diseases concurrently which will complicate nursing care. Knowledge of social problems will help a nurse to plan for discharge. The student will learn more effectively through identifying the particular needs and problems of each patient. The formulation of care plans is a valuable teaching and learning exercise, provided the student has guidance from an experienced member of staff. Planning care also requires a sound understanding of the pathology of the patient's illness, the clinical features produced, and the appropriate medical treatment. After a full assessment, priorities of care can be determined from both the nurse's and the patient's perspective.

As already mentioned, the learner requires support and guidance, not only in the formulation of a care plan, but also in the implementation of care.

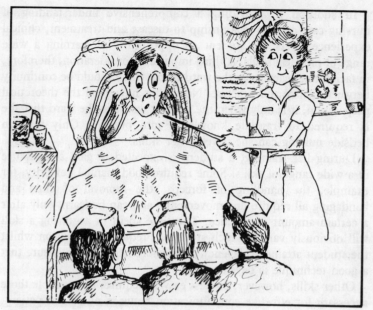

Fig. 3.1

It has been emphasised that the learner needs support and guidance when carrying out new skills. Team nursing not only provides this support but offers a way in which the fullest value can be gained from the opportunities for ward learning. Under this system, junior and senior nurses work closely together in the care of a group of patients. The team is accountable to the ward sister, and some overall supervision will be necessary. But otherwise the team organises and implements the nursing care, and carries full responsibility for the group of patients. Some care needs to be carried out by two nurses, and the less experienced will learn from the other. Provided the example set is good, the student will learn not only about the physical care of the patient but also about his psychological needs. The junior will observe an experienced nurse explaining investigations, comforting bereaved relatives or communicating with a deaf patient. At the same time, the senior nurse in the team can learn the importance of planning and organisation, and the need to give clear and accurate instructions about patient care. Each member of the team will learn to contribute, develop initiative and gain a sense of responsibility. Teaching and learning will become a joint effort between junior and senior learners. Team nursing in the ward provides a preparation for the staff nurse's role, which otherwise may be neglected in nurse training.

In addition to providing a comprehensive understanding of nursing care and its relationship to disease and treatment, clinical experience offers the student an opportunity of learning a wide range of practical skills. A third important consideration, therefore, in facilitating learning in the ward is that there should be continuity between theory and practice. No matter how good the theoretical preparation, it is only when the student works in the ward that she is required to translate knowledge into practice. Only through bedside nursing can she develop her skills.

During her training, a student is expected to gain competence in a wide range of skills. Some require good manual dexterity, for example, the handling of forceps, the removal of clips and bandaging all require fine movements, and can be learnt only after a certain amount of practice. The time spent in acquiring a skill will obviously vary for each student. Frequent supervision whilst the student attains proficiency is therefore necessary to ensure that a good technique is developed.

Other skills, however, are less easy to acquire, for example those necessary for effective communication between nurse and patient. The planning of each patient's care is dependent upon a comprehensive and accurate assessment. A lot of the necessary information is obtained through discussion with the patient and his relatives.

A student can learn much about interpersonal skills through observation of more experienced staff. Through the application of her knowledge of theories of interaction, the student will learn to develop constructive relationships with patients.

Some preparation in nursing care and skills is obviously necessary before the full benefit of learning at the bedside can be derived. Classroom instruction is invaluable in providing some of this background and in giving the learner confidence. Textbooks are also useful, but have their limitations. Diseases are categorised and insufficient note is made of the effect of multiple pathology on the problems of the patient. The information in textbooks also becomes outdated quickly, and therefore details of recent research and developments are not always included. Computer-aided learning is still in its infancy in nurse education, but (as with textbooks) this method of learning can only help the student to acquire knowledge, not practical experience.

Problems may occur when the sequence of learning in the school does not correspond to clinical practice. There may be a time lapse between teaching and practical experience, so that recall may be impaired. Hence the excuse often heard from a student 'But I am sure that I learnt that in the school!' The modular system, whereby the theory and practice of a particular specialty are co-ordinated, has done much to minimise these problems. The learner, however, is still frequently confronted by the unfamiliar. As well as encouraging her to apply general known principles, the ward staff also need to provide tuition and support. This brings us to another important point. Teaching in the classroom and on the ward must correspond. On the one hand, there is no value in tutorial staff teaching unrealistic and out-of-date care which the learner has to unlearn in the ward. On the other hand, the ward staff should adopt a uniform standard and method throughout the hospital. This practice should be based on proven principles, acceptable to all, and not on routine and ritual.

Classroom teaching is therefore important in helping the student to develop confidence and competence. The student's understanding of the wide range of topics taught will be tested only when she is required to put it into practice. There are some interesting observations about this in Eve Bendall's study 'So you passed, nurse' (Bendall 1975).

The ward thus provides an ideal setting for learning. But the student must also be encouraged to learn, and be helped to recognise opportunities for doing so. Students often complain that nothing has been learned from a particular allocation. This may be because no formal teaching sessions took place, and no specific assessment of skills occurred. Ward learning is however a gradual process, and the student can easily overlook the value of discussions of patients' progress, the care supervised by a senior nurse and the opportunity to observe experienced people at work. Teaching and learning are very different, and the student must not rely on teaching alone for development of expertise. Ward objectives will give her guidance in making the most of each allocation.

Some of the problems

There are obviously going to be problems associated with learning at the bedside. The organisation of a ward is directed towards ensuring the best possible standard of patient care, and is not primarily concerned with the needs of the learner. A conflict between service demands and educational requirements can occur. However, the teaching of students is a necessary prerequisite of good patient care. Some of the problems that arise cannot be solved immediately, but in the long term many can be anticipated and overcome.

The ward is not a classroom, and teaching and learning cannot take place without interruptions and constraints. In the school, teaching takes place in purpose-built or adapted classrooms where equipment is plentiful and space adequate. Reality strikes home when the learner arrives on the ward to find it overcrowded with beds, chairs, trolleys and even patients. Skills have to be exercised in a cramped space amid the noise and activity of the ward. Teaching and supervision may be interrupted by the unexpected, making concentration and learning difficult. This, however, is the reality of nursing, and the student must be helped to adapt to all situations.

Despite good management on the ward, there are always times when some equipment is lacking. But the absence, say, of sterile dressing packs can be turned to good use. The student has to improvise and adapt the procedure without departing from the principles of aseptic technique. The way in which she copes is a real test of her understanding.

Lack of time is a perpetual problem for the ward staff and may be given as an excuse for the failure of ward teaching and supervision. Teaching does indeed take time, but in the long term it is a great time saver. A learner who lacks confidence and competence will take much longer to implement care, and will also put the patient at risk. Poor techniques will develop, and these may be passed on to more junior learners. Substandard nursing practice may or may not be the fault of the individual, but it always points to inadequate supervision and teaching. Opportunities for teaching occur spontaneously throughout every day, and do not need to be manufactured or to be time consuming. These will be discussed later.

It is impossible to predict bed occupancy, or to some extent, the types of patient who will be admitted at various times of the year. An orthopaedic and trauma admission ward is a good example of this. Emergency admissions as a result of road traffic accidents or falls on icy pavements cannot be arranged. The student may nurse only patients with ingrowing toe nails or hallux valgus. The resulting clinical experience is limited, and not fully representative of the specialty. The ward staff, however, can provide additional practical experience to compensate. For example, observation in a fracture clinic or operating theatre can be arranged. Suitable ward-based projects give the student opportunities to set up traction or to practise orthopaedic procedures. Although these situations are contrived, the learner gains valuable experience in the care of patients with orthopaedic problems.

Staffing levels are also difficult to predict, and holidays or sickness may leave a ward very short of nurses, both trained and untrained. In these circumstances, the senior staff will find it virtually impossible to teach and supervise students as well as provide the patients with adequate nursing care. Some degree of 'task allocation' may become necessary, though the concept of total patient care should never be completely abandoned. By good planning and communication, the identification of priority tasks and their allocation among the members of the team, the learner is helped to work efficiently and effectively. The students will benefit by gaining insight into the importance of communication and organisation, and will learn how to adapt to different environments.

No one can predict when a busy period may occur in the ward. Therefore any available time during less busy periods should be used for teaching. In this way, the learner will gain confidence, and this goes a long way to promoting safe practice if at a later time adequate guidance and support are lacking.

As most of the ward learning occurs at the bedside, full discussion of the patient and his treatment provides another problem. Whenever possible, the patient should be included in discussions about his care. A separate venue must be available, however, if confidential information is to be considered in relation to nursing care. Free discussion about the quality of the work of the learner is also necessary, and is best done away from the bedside. This follow-up is essential in ward teaching, but poor facilities often make it difficult to achieve without interruption.

A ward full of learning opportunities does not automatically ensure that the student will learn. She may lack motivation to increase knowledge and improve skills, and appear uninterested. This attitude often hides a fear of failing or of making mistakes. Lack of support during previous clinical experience may have sapped the confidence of the learner. During training the student will learn from many teachers, and the junior nurse can be confused by apparent differences and contradictions. Each teacher approaches a procedure in an individual way and has different areas of expertise and interest. Similarly, each teacher will make different demands on the learner, and variable standards may be expected. As the nurse becomes more experienced, the material taught can be evaluated, but the junior nurse may become muddled and feel insecure. The ward staff should be aware of this problem and give extra support and supervision when necessary.

The student may also appear uninterested because of a lack of job satisfaction and encouragement. Actual dislike of a specialty will produce a negative student who does not want to learn. Recognition of good work carried out by a student and help in improving standards when her work is less good will demonstrate the interest of the ward staff in her progress. This will help to promote interest and motivation to learn. The senior staff also need to be alert to other problems, such as illness and personal worries which interfere with learning. This is not only in the interests of the student but also helps to ensure a good standard of nursing.

As mentioned earlier, the needs of the patient are always of prime importance in nursing care, and teaching must not interfere with this care. Unnecessary procedures must never be carried out just because a learner needs the practice. But it should be possible by careful organisation to arrange both that the patient gets the best care, and that the learner gains the experience she needs. Care can, for example, be timed so that a particular nurse has the chance to develop the skills she lacks. Allocation of work using total patient care should secure this, but as the patient's needs are constantly changing it may not always succeed.

The ward is thus a ready-made learning resource centre with the facilities and staff to promote the development of good nursing care by the student. But as with any organisation, it is not without problems and these can hinder its effectiveness. The permanent ward staff bear the responsibility for finding ways to overcome or minimise these problems, so as to enable the ward to play its full part in the training programme. At the same time, the learner must be encouraged to take every opportunity both to learn and to participate in the teaching of others.

Resources for ward learning

A later chapter will discuss in full the use of audio-visual aids in ward learning. But brief mention of them will be made here as the opportunities for ward learning are so greatly enhanced by the provision of appropriate resources. Questions can be answered as they arise, and spare time can be used to broaden understanding of a diagnosis or treatment. The information can be presented in different forms.

Reference books can form the basis of a small library. These should be selected by the ward sister and school of nursing librarian so that the particular specialities of the ward are covered. As finance for books may be limited, money given by patients could be used for this purpose. Some books will no doubt disappear, but this should not lead to the library being discontinued.

The provision of learning resources need not be costly, as many drug firms provide information free. It is possible for the ward to collect and develop its own material. Articles from the nursing press and newspapers and ward-made charts will supplement the library. Copies of interesting x-rays or photographs can be kept, thus further increasing learning resources. Large clear diagrams drawn on sugar paper and covered with transparent film are particularly useful teaching aids. They are also invaluable when explaining treatment to patients and relatives. Students should be encouraged to produce their own teaching material. This not only augments the supply of visual aids, but is an excellent method of learning.

Each ward should have written guidelines on how to undertake procedures. Staff can produce an individual handbook covering specific aspects of care, for example pre-operative preparation or a doctor's preferences for treatment. This is particularly helpful to the student at the beginning of her allocation. It is important, however, that the information is not presented in such a way as to perpetuate routine and ritual. Whenever possible, the reason for the recommended method should be given.

Other information which should be readily available to the learner includes nursing records. These must be written legibly and without abbreviation, so that the student can make maximum use of them. Understanding of the total care of a patient is not helped by references such as S.O.B., N.B.M. or T.L.C. In addition, the care plans and progress notes are professional records. Although queries and complaints are relatively few, a comprehensive record is vital if legal action is taken. The solicitor's defence is only a good as the quality of the information in the written documents.

Medical records are also useful in helping the student to learn about all aspects of a patient's care. The value of a doctor's notes is greatly enhanced if the information is concisely presented. Problem-orientated medical records (POMR) are now used by many doctors. This system, devised by Weed (1969) complements the problem-solving approach used in nursing care planning.

Information of current interest or related to the ward learning programme can be presented in a display form. A notice board placed in a suitable part of the ward is useful for presenting learning material. Responsibility for changing this and keeping information up to date can be delegated to a staff nurse or senior student.

Students will have an incentive to seek more information about the patient if the information is well presented. Material should also be selected carefully as the quality of the resource is more important than the quantity. An immense pile of out-of-date articles will possibly obscure the purpose in view and deter the student from learning.

The teachers in the ward

Students have been vocal in recent years about the lack of supervision and support in the wards. As stressed earlier, inadequate guidance when new nursing skills are performed causes anxiety, not only to the learner but also the patient. This leads to job dissatisfaction for the learner and can adversely influence the recovery of the patient. Yet constant supervision and guidance would be costly in personnel and could retard the development of independence and initiative in the learner.

All trained staff in the clinical field have a responsibility to teach, although few will have had formal preparation for this. The permanent ward staff are in the best position to encourage learning. They are the experts in the care of the types of patients admitted to the ward, and are familiar with the specific skills, routines and demands. They also provide a stable focus around which the ward organisation revolves. It is in the interest of the senior staff to ensure that the best nursing care is given, and that the learner is safe and reliable. This automatically necessitates teaching and supervision. There is, however, a conflict between teaching and the many other commitments to the ward. The senior staff have many competing responsibilities. Overall supervision of a ward is in itself a mammoth task and constant interruptions make the concentration on one patient or learner difficult.

The geography of the modern hospital has also brought problems. In the Nightingale Ward, the sister could see the beds, patients and learners from one place and quickly assess the situation. The small unit arrangement, although more intimate for the patient, has meant detachment for the nurse-in-charge. It is now necessary to walk much further to see the patients, and a nurse or patient in trouble may not be immediately detected. Curtains around a bed can also hide a multitude of sins in patient care. The learner who apparently works quickly and efficiently may have much to learn in bedside nursing. It would be impossible to supervise everyone, but nursing care must be monitored to prevent substandard practice developing.

Few of the trained staff have had any guidance in how to teach, and this may produce a feeling of inadequacy. Not everyone wants to teach, and with the very rapid advances in treatment the ward sister may sometimes have an uneasy feeling that the student is more up-to-date than she herself. Confidence can be obtained from further education. The past few years have seen the development of continuing education programmes for trained staff. It has been appreciated that learning does not stop with the examinations for registrations. Some post-basic courses (such as the English National Board Clinical Courses and the Diploma in Nursing) have curricula leading to a recognised qualification. Other courses have developed on an ad hoc basis to meet the learning requirements of trained nurses. Excellent study days and short courses on ward teaching are now being arranged in some Schools of Nursing. These provide an opportunity for ward staff to obtain guidance on how best to pass on their clinical expertise in an effective way.

Despite the problems, the trained ward staff are in an ideal situation to guide the learner in her development of nursing skills. They can detect problems which may hinder learning. If there is a good relationship within the ward team, the student will feel able to discuss difficulties as they arise. She will also feel able to draw on the great assets the team have to offer, namely experience and a wide knowledge of patient care.

Senior students too are valuable teachers in the ward team. Preparation for instruction is again minimal, but with help from the trained staff the senior learner can develop a teaching role. This secures extra teaching for the junior nurse, and the senior student will herself learn from this role. She will gain confidence in communication and management skills, and her own knowledge will be tested. It is well known that one of the best ways of learning is to teach others. The student 'teacher' will have a responsibility to maintain standards, and this should be reflected in an improvement in her own nursing skills. The more senior nurse can also support the junior in difficult situations because of her own recent experience. The ward sister and trained staff on the other hand may have forgotten the small incidents which cause anxiety in the learner.

The junior nurse should also be involved in teaching. The sequence of clinical allocations is such that the junior may have more experience in a particular area than a senior student. Seniority does not necessarily denote competence in all procedures. The senior learner should not feel ashamed if in some things a junior is more skilled. Everyone has a contribution to make to ward teaching and the student should take every possible opportunity to learn.

The senior nurse should participate in the teaching of students in the unit. Again this is not her prime responsibility and preparation for teaching may be limited. But in her routine work there is ample opportunity for teaching. The daily visit to a ward provides an opportunity for hearing a report on the patients from the learner. This can be used as a teaching session while providing the senior nurse with some of the information required for the management of the unit. The senior nurse may also allocate time for individual teaching of learners, or for group tutorial sessions. Her contribution in discussion of ward management will be particularly relevant and useful.

A clinical nurse specialist, such as the stoma therapist, is also invaluable in the teaching of students. The role of the specialist must include teaching the nurse as well as the patient. Thus her expertise is passed on. Education of all the ward team promotes continuity in the specialised care of the patient and increases the skill of the nurse.

Other specialists too, such as those in the paramedical field, may be involved in ward teaching. The physiotherapist, dietitian or hospital chaplain should explain and discuss their contributions to the total care of the patient. Community aspects of care must also be included, so that the learner understands the importance of both hospital and home. Cooperation between all concerned with patient care will be improved when the function of each role is discussed and understood. Where appropriate, paramedical staff should be asked to participate in ward tutorials. For example, a tutorial about abortion would obviously include some discussion about the ethical aspects of therapeutic abortion. This can be made more valuable by the inclusion of the hospital chaplain.

The student can also learn about the role of other members of the ward team by visits to departments such as the diet kitchen or occupational therapy unit. Whenever possible, students should have the opportunity of accompanying the occupational therapist or physiotherapist on a home visit. The learner will thereby gain a much greater understanding of the patient. This should at the same time lead to improved continuity of care for the patient.

The medical staff can help directly and indirectly in the teaching of students. By recognising the complexity of the work of the ward sister and the demands made on her time, doctors can help by co-operating in good ward management. Planning of ward rounds and non-urgent procedures in conjunction with the nurse-in-charge leads to better organisation. Learners should participate in ward rounds and medical procedures, and accompany the doctor when a patient is being examined. If total patient care is practised, the learner is able to report her observations on the progress of the patient and learn first-hand about future care. The reasons for treatment, the purpose of investigations and the progress of the patient can be discussed with the doctor.

The doctor can also help by writing comprehensive and legible medical notes. Information and instructions are often misunderstood or misinterpreted because of illegibility or abbreviation. The ward sister and doctor may be able to formulate a medical examination sheet. This can be designed to include problem-orientated recording, the system outlined earlier in the chapter. The introduction of a pre-printed form will save medical staff time as well as aid student learning.

So far, the personnel mentioned in relation to ward teaching are those with little or no specific preparation for it. Some are natural teachers and enjoy this role, drawing on a wealth of experience. The tutor and the clinical teacher, on the other hand, have had specific preparation for teaching, and therefore have a well-defined part to play in ward teaching.

The registered nurse tutor is involved in the education of the learner throughout training, and has a heavy commitment to teaching in the school of nursing. Preparation for classes, actual teaching and administrative duties necessarily limit the time available to her for bedside teaching. Nonetheless, most tutors are involved in some way with ward learning. The ward may be used in conjunction with a classroom session, patient care being used to demonstrate the practical application of a particular subject. Furthermore, the tutor may be allocated to a particular ward or unit to help to co-ordinate the learning programme. She can advise on ward objectives, teaching content and methods of presentation. She may also participate in the ward teaching, either at the bedside or by leading tutorial sessions. The learner benefits from the extra supervision and teaching, and the tutor is able to assess the student's progress in practical skills. The tutor can also keep up with developments in treatment and patient care, and is made aware of the stresses these may put on the learners. The ward staff, too, benefit from the addition of a trained nurse, one who is able to teach students patient care and relieve them of some of this responsibility. Indeed, in some hospitals, joint appointments of ward sister and teacher have been introduced. By alternating the two roles, the appointee provides an invaluable link between clinical practice and theory, and between service and school of nursing.

The role of the clinical teacher has been discussed in the previous chapter. Here, therefore, only the opportunities and problems in bedside nursing as they affect the clinical teacher will be mentioned.

The clinical teacher is involved not only in the education of the learner and the care of the patient, but also in the maintenance of good relationships and communication between the ward and the school of nursing. She has a highly interesting job which allows her to remain in close contact with patient care. She also has the added stimulus of teaching.

The work of the clinical teacher is influenced by the way in which her responsibilities are organised. She may be allocated a group of learners, and follow them throughout their training. This means that the clinical teacher has to work in many different wards. Alternatively, she may be allocated specific wards where she is responsible for all learners who work there. Both systems have advantages and disadvantages.

Supervising a group of learners throughout the whole of their training is very satisfying for the clinical teacher. She can maintain individual contact and watch the progress of the students. The teacher and student get to know each other well, and therefore work in a relaxed productive way. The needs of each learner will be recognised and work can be planned to meet them. Where there is a personality clash, the learner should be re-allocated to another clinical teacher. For her part, however, the clinical teacher has to work in many wards, and is unable to become expert in any one speciality. Contact with the ward staff and the patients will be short and will lack continuity. As a result, good relationships are hard to build up and maintain.

Allocation to specific wards allows the clinical teacher and ward staff to work closely together to improve learning opportunities for the student. The clinical teacher can become knowledgeable about a particular specialty, and will be aware of the demands of the ward. She will know the stage reached in the care of each of the patients and will be able to establish a good relationship with them.

The drawback of this system is that the clinical teacher works only briefly with each student and has little on which to assess progress. She can find herself working exclusively with the obvious problem students. Good and less good students all need teaching and supervision in their clinical work. Yet it is often the students who have failed an assessment who receive most attention.

The clinical teacher must have a good method of communicating the progress of the learner to ward staff and tutor. She does not work in isolation, and poor records will deprive others involved in teaching of vital information about the student.

The work of the clinical teacher is based on relationships, and the success or failure of these relationships will affect her efficiency and effectiveness. It is the responsibility of the clinical teacher to ensure that everyone understands her role and the important part she plays in nurse education. Too often the role is not understood, and she is in danger of becoming a general factotum (Fig. 3.2).

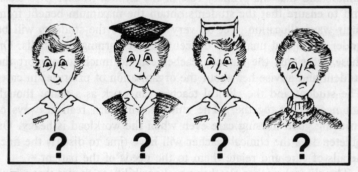

Fig. 3.2

Firstly, the clinical teacher must have a good relationship with the staff of the school of nursing. The major part of her work is in the instruction of learners. Policies affecting nurse education will therefore influence this work. It is unfortunate that a clinical teacher may not always be involved in decisions taken by the school. The clinical teacher can make a valuable contribution, and nurse education benefits when tutors and clinical teachers work closely together.

The clinical teacher must also be involved in planning time-tables, since she is often required to teach in the classroom. Ward teaching commitments must be honoured, and this cannot be done if the clinical teacher is asked at short notice to participate in class-room teaching. Sensible planning and co-operation will minimise the time spent away from the ward; for example, sessions in the school from 10 a.m. to 11 a.m. make ward teaching difficult.

Secondly, the clinical teacher should establish good relationships with the ward sister and staff. She must respect the ideas and methods of the ward, provided of course that these correspond to accepted hospital practice. A good spirit of understanding between the ward staff and the clinical teacher makes the task of ward teaching much easier. Too often the clinical teacher is looked upon as an interfering and critical representative of the school of nursing – and as one who takes three hours to teach a student how to take a blood pressure! The truth is that learning new skills does take time, and progress may appear to be very slow. In the long term, however, the ward benefits from a student who through supervision becomes more competent in the care she gives.

The clinical teacher should be part of the ward team, but must resist becoming an extra pair of hands. The ward staff should understand that the primary role of the clinical teacher is to teach and to ensure that the students obtain the maximum benefit from their ward allocation. Yet on very busy days the students will be under stress and unable to concentrate on learning new skills. On these occasions, the clinical teacher can do much to support the student and advise her about the organisation of priorities in care. The student and the clinical teacher can work as a team, though not necessarily together. The student will learn realistic ways of ensuring good nursing care even when the workload is heavy. On quieter days the clinical teacher will have time to discuss the finer details of care and relate them to the needs of the patient.

The clinical teacher also has a responsibility to ensure that a high standard of nursing care is given to the patient. This must, however, be done in a realistic and sensible way, the demands of the ward being balanced with the needs of the learner. To ask, without prior notice, to withdraw six students for a tutorial when the ward is desperately busy will not help relationships.

Thirdly, the clinical teacher must develop a good relationship with the learner. This is a priority because a tense, nervous student will not work well, and will be unresponsive to teaching. The clinical teacher is not a highly critical 'examiner', as the student sometimes thinks. She and the learner should work together, as partners, to achieve a high standard of care. The teacher, while not allowing poor practice, needs to remember that the learner is a learner and needs the opportunity to become proficient. On the other hand, the student must not be spoon-fed. She should be encouraged to take the initiative in solving problems of care, always with the sympathetic support of the clinical teacher.

The clinical teacher has another role, as counsellor to the learner. She is involved in clinical nursing, yet is detached from the ward team. If a good relationship exists, the student should feel able to discuss anxieties and problems which may interfere with learning. For this purpose, it is essential that the clinical teacher has access to a room where discussion can be private and uninterrupted.

Finally, the clinical teacher has to maintain a good relationship with patients and relatives. She may be dressed in a different uniform, and therefore must explain her role to the patient. For effective teaching, the confidence and co-operation of the patient are essential. Patients often feel a responsibility for junior nurses and may resent the intrusion of another person whose presence inhibits their relationship with the learners. When one carries out patient care, one must always remember that the needs of the patient take precedence over the needs of the learner. Clinical teaching with a relaxed learner and patient can be great fun, and all three can learn from each other.

Because the clinical teacher works in both the ward and the school, there is a danger that she becomes part of neither. She has a commitment to both, and may be torn between the two. She cannot readily down tools during the resuscitation of a patient to be on time at a meeting in the school. On the other hand, the ward may not understand the demands made by the school. Non-appearance on the ward does not necessarily mean that the clinical teacher has overslept or is sitting, feet up, drinking cups of tea. To fulfil her role properly, she must have time to prepare sessions and keep up to date with a wide range of subjects.

Despite many problems, the work of a clinical teacher is immensely rewarding. It can be very tiring, and she has to adapt constantly to the changing needs of the learner, patient and ward. The job is what the individual makes it, and the onus is on the clinical teacher to explain her role and ensure that it is recognised by all. This positive approach brings benefits which contribute greatly to the improvement of ward learning. It is then up to the clinical teacher to check the effectiveness of her own work by watching the students' progress in attaining a high standard of nursing care.

Ward learning and the ward sister

The previous section has outlined the contribution made by the clinical teacher to ward teaching and learning. The success of her work, however, is dependent upon her relationships with the ward team. Central to this team is the ward sister, and she is the key to creating a good learning environment. The findings of current research into the role of the ward sister highlight her importance. In particular, her leadership influences the type of ward management and 'atmosphere'.

Pembrey (1980), in her study of the role of the ward sister, looked at the management cycle in relation to the organisation of nursing care. The good ward manager took into account the individual requirements of both patient and nurse when organising care. These management skills had been learnt through observation of other sisters rather than from formal management courses.

The style of ward sister leadership was explored further by Ogier (1982). She observed the verbal interactions between sister and learner. She also elicited the views of the students about the way ward organisation helped them to learn. Highly rated were sisters who were approachable, oriented to nurse learners, and who gave explicit directions about nursing care. Interestingly, however, Ogier found that the 'ideal' sister may have different characteristics, depending on the speciality of the ward.

Fretwell (1982) studied in more detail the clinical learning environment. She contended that, although on paper two wards might appear very similar, there were considerable differences in the experience offered to students. She observed that sisters have different management styles and ward routines which contribute to a variation in ward 'atmosphere'. She says 'It was clear that the sister's influence on learning extended beyond the actual teaching she did; for she was able to initiate teaching and (through her ward organisation) place learners in situations in which they had an opportunity to learn' (Fretwell, 1980, p. 70).

The amount of time spent by ward sisters on teaching varies considerably. Sisters were categorised by Orton (1980) as having either a high or a low student orientation. 'Orientation' described the sister's attitude and behaviour towards learners on her ward. Sisters with a high orientation were found to spend on average 16% of their time teaching, whereas those with a low orientation spent 11%. She concludes from her study that there is strong evidence to suggest that the ward 'climate' is an important factor in the satisfaction of students with their learning environment.

An evaluation of the ward as a learning environment will be completed by 1986 by researchers at the Nursing Education

Research Unit, Chelsea College. Results of the pilot study (Lewin and Leach 1982) indicate some of the characteristics of a 'good' ward. Although the time spent teaching was said to be similar on most wards, the trained staff on a good ward devoted more time to supervision, practical demonstrations and participation in ward reporting sessions.

The findings from these research projects are obviously important for ward learning and teaching. The links between the characteristics of the ward sister, her management style and the provision of clinical experience for learners are clearly demonstrated. The ideal sister is democratic, patient-orientated, and fulfils an active teaching role. It might seem that good ward sisters are made in heaven! The results of the research projects, however, do have practical implications for the selection and training of sisters.

Preparation for the role of the ward sister has been haphazard. In the past, a new sister has learned mainly through observation of those more experienced; and then, through trial and error, has developed her own style of ward management. As discussed earlier in the chapter, there are increasing opportunities for continuing education for trained nurses. Formal education, however, may not be enough. Pembrey's findings were that the role model was important in helping a sister to develop a good management style. This conclusion was the main impetus behind the King's Fund scheme of ward training for newly appointed sisters. The experiment has been described by Hazel Allen (1982).

As the complexity of the work of a ward sister grows, it is important that her contribution to ward teaching is not lost. Although the time she spends actively involved in teaching may be limited, she can, through her organisation of nursing care, facilitate teaching by others.

Assessing the learning requirements and progress of students

As outlined at the beginning of the chapter, for the student to make full use of the learning opportunities available during a ward allocation she must be aware of what these are. Similarly, the ward sister must know the previous experience of the learner, what her capabilities are and what she needs to learn on the ward.

An introductory letter can be sent to the learner before the allocation starts (Table 3.1). This will introduce the student to the speciality of the ward, and give her time for preparation. The letter

Table 3.1

Ward A
Telephone Number
Date

Dear Nurse _____,
    You have been assigned to Ward A, commencing on _____.
    Ward A is part of the Surgical Unit and has 26 beds. The main
specialty is gynaecology. The ward nursing staff are all willing to help
and supervise you during your allocation. They are:
    Ward Sister – Miss B.
    2 Staff Nurses and 1 Enrolled Nurse.
    Senior Nurse – Miss C.
    and Clinical Teacher – Miss D.
There are many opportunities to learn, and we hope you will make full
use of the ward programme. A copy of the ward learning objectives and
teaching programme is enclosed.
    Before you start your clinical experience, you are advised to revise the
anatomy and physiology of the female genito-urinary tract. This will
help in your understanding of your patients and their care.
    If you have any off-duty requests or queries please contact us.
    We look forward to working with you.
        Yours sincerely,

        _____

---

also removes some of the fear of the unknown, and will help the
learner to settle more quickly. On arrival, the ward sister and
learner should have a preliminary discussion. The ward sister can
explain what she expects the nurse to learn during the allocation,
and can set objectives. The ward teaching programme can be
explained, and the learner shown the ward learning resources. The
ward sister also must establish the needs of the student, and how
best to meet them. Actual nursing practice can only be assessed
in the ward, so supervision and teaching must be organised. The
student may have particular needs. For example, she may be
required to take an assessment of her nursing skills for examination
purposes during the allocation, and may need extra help for this
purpose. The assessment should not trigger off frantic practising,
but the ward sister can arrange for the student to have the relevant
experience. Where continuous assessment of clinical competence
is used, the ward sister and student can outline their aims for the
allocation.

    This first discussion will demonstrate to the student the interest
of the ward staff in her and in her progress. She will feel accepted
as a member of the ward team and will be more ready to learn.
Opportunities for valuable experience will not be wasted, as both
ward sister and learner are aware of what needs to be achieved.

Follow-up discussion is equally important, as the student needs to know how she is progressing. This can occur at any time but particularly when the student has been observed or supervised in her nursing care. An accurate record of her progress needs to be kept and a check made on the experience she has gained. An assessment of progress is essential midway through the allocation. The student will then have time to act on the report, and the ward sister will then be able to evaluate the ward teaching and rectify omissions in the student's experience.

The final discussion will include evaluation of the ward learning programme by the student. This will help the ward staff to improve teaching content and methods. The ward sister will be required to write a ward report on the student, and this must be discussed fully with her. Testing of knowledge gained can be centred around the ward learning objectives. The student may have submitted written work or completed work sheets while on the ward, and these should be marked and returned.

These discussions take time but are essential to ward teaching. The students and her needs must be known to the ward staff if learning is to be effective. Too often the student and her capabilities are matched to the number of stars and stripes she has on her uniform. Similarly the student must be aware of the opportunities for learning, so that she is able to make full use of her time on the ward.

Teaching opportunities in the ward

Earlier in the chapter it was mentioned that there are many ways in which teaching and learning can be incorporated in the normal routine of the ward. During an allocation, the student will acquire new knowledge and skills, most of which will be learned in an informal and unstructured way. The requirements of each learner are different, and the ways in which she learns best also differ. One student will gain more from one method of teaching than from another.

The opportunities for the education of the student during her ward allocation must not be left to chance. Each ward should have a planned programme which makes full use of its learning opportunities. The overall responsibility for the organisation of the ward learning programme can be delegated to one particular member of staff, but everyone in the ward team should participate. Teaching methods will take various forms.

The role model

Teaching by example can be one of the best ways of passing on skills, provided of course that the example is good. Students are observing all the time the nursing care given by others, so the senior staff are in an ideal position to demonstrate good care. This will include practical skills, organisation, communication and also attitudes to patients.

An experienced nurse should demonstrate a new nursing skill before the learner attempts it herself. A high standard set by the skilled nurse should be reflected in the performance of the learner. The student should be critical of everything observed, as blind acceptance is dangerous. This is particularly so if the standard of care is bad, because poor nursing care will then be perpetuated. Students observing poor nursing care will find it difficult to maintain good standards themselves. The learner may even be ridiculed for taking too long in her care, and an attitude of 'why bother?' will develop. This is obviously not conducive to ward learning, and valuable clinical experience is wasted.

Attitudes to patient care can be passed from the ward staff to the learner. The ward sister who spends time talking to the patients and is interested in them as individuals will pass this approach on to the junior nurse. The student will not feel a sense of guilt if she sits down to talk to an anxious patient. The attitude of the learner to the patient can also be adversely affected by what is said. A senior nurse who describes a patient as 'difficult' or 'demanding' will influence the way in which the others view the patient. This is well illustrated in *The Unpopular Patient* (1972) by Felicity Stockwell.

The quality of ward organisation and communication is also reflected in the learner's performance. The student will learn from experience about the importance of planning, and passing on information. A chaotic ward, where no instructions are given about patient care, will usually result in bad nursing care. The student is unable to work methodically and priorities cannot be set. It is true that some nurses who observe poor standards in ward management or patient care will resolve never to perform so badly. Learning is therefore achieved in a negative way, but a certain amount of experience is necessary before such an evaluation can be made.

Both junior and senior nurses and others involved in patient care can be the 'model' from which the learning occurs. When working together in a team, the members can learn much from each other. If one of them is aware that she is providing an example for the others, she will have an additional incentive to set a high standard. Every nurse in the ward is responsible for promoting good nursing care. This can easily be achieved if teaching by example is recognised as a valuable way of passing on expertise.

Individual teaching and supervision

One of the most intensive ways in which a student can learn at the bedside is from individual tuition. The teacher may be a more experienced student, one of the ward's trained staff or the clinical teacher. The learner works closely with her instructor while carrying out nursing care. This type of teaching has obvious benefits for the learner because her special needs can be met. The teacher can concentrate on improving particular aspects of the student's skills.

All opportunities that arise for one-to-one teaching should be taken. As in teaching by example, special arrangements do not need to be made for individual supervision. For example, two nurses are required to do the medicine round, and the administration of drugs can be used as a learning opportunity. The senior nurse will ensure that the learner is checking and giving drugs in the correct way. As the drugs are checked, the learner's knowledge of the action and side effects can be tested. The administration of the medications can then be related to the patient and the treatment of disease; the student is learning not only safety in drug administration, but also more about the total care of patients. Another opportunity for individual teaching occurs when the learner acts as assistant for a clinical procedure. In this situation the teacher could be a doctor, physiotherapist or clinical nurse specialist. The student will have an opportunity to observe and ask questions. As well as acting as a support for the patient she will be gaining additional information relevant to her understanding of patient care.

The learner can be taught when she reports to the ward sister and other members of the nursing team about the care and progress of her patients. Discussion of the problems and treatment of each patient in relation to nursing care planned will help ensure that the learner understands the rationale for such care. The student's observation of a patient will be tested, and she can be guided to evaluate her work. Short sessions such as these are invaluable as the student is learning from actual patient care, and a wide range of subjects will be drawn together in order to bring about better understanding of this care.

Although these opportunities for learning occur within the framework of the ward's routine, extra time will be needed if student tuition is included. The teacher may feel it is quicker and less tiring to carry out the task alone, or to ignore teaching opportunities. But this defeats the idea of ward learning, and the students will suffer in their development of knowledge and skills.

A more structured approach to one-to-one teaching occurs when someone, for example the clinical teacher, arranges to work with a learner on a specific day. The session is discussed beforehand with the student so that her particular needs are met. Objectives for learning can be set so that the nurse has guidelines for the session. Where possible, the clinical teacher arranges for the ward staff to allocate patient care to provide the best experience for the learner in this supervised role.

Learning should be centred around the total care of a group of patients. The responsibility for planning their care should be with the learner. Problem solving is invaluable in increasing the learner's adaptability and confidence. The clinical teacher can guide and advise but should never monopolise the situation. There should be time not only to carry out the patient care but also to discuss and evaluate it. Therefore the work load should not be too heavy.

The value of this type of teaching is immense. There is an opportunity to relate theory to practice, and as the teaching is set at the student's level of understanding and experience, time can be spent on aspects which she finds difficult. Practical skills will be included and new experience will be gained under supervision.

One-to-one teaching is tiring for both learner and teacher, as the session requires a high degree of concentration from both. The teacher must ensure that the student is relaxed, so that stress does not interfere with learning. If the session is viewed as a dreaded ordeal, the learner will feel anxious and not gain maximum benefit. Overteaching must be avoided as the learner will become confused and end up by remembering nothing. Important points should be emphasised and reinforced. Guidance about further reading can be given so that learning continues and is not viewed as a once and for all matter.

The clinical teacher must be adaptable, as the objectives set for the student may need to be revised because of altered patient care.

For example, the scheduled removal of sutures from a patient's wound may be delayed because of poor healing. But catheterisation may become necessary because the patient develops retention of urine. Here the needs of the patient obviously override the needs of the learner. This situation is a reminder that no two patients are the same, and that the learner must be adaptable in the nursing care she gives.

While teaching, whether in a structured or unstructured way, the teacher will get to know the learners and their individual weaknesses and strengths. The students must have full information about performance – including both praise and criticism. An honest appraisal will help their progress and guide them to further learning opportunities.

Group teaching

There are many situations when learning on the ward is better achieved in groups. This method is less time-consuming as one teacher will be teaching several learners. As with individual teaching, group teaching can be structured or unstructured.

The ward report on the progress of each patient, which is given at the beginning of a shift, is an example of group teaching that can be given in the normal routine of the ward.

Full discussion will lead to a better understanding of the patient. The ward sister has up-to-date information, for example, the social worker's reports or changes in treatment. The student will have been in close contact with the patient while carrying out nursing care, and will have observed the patient's progress. All information can be pooled at the report session, and problems discussed and clarified. The active participation of the learner should be encouraged as this will lead to improved confidence and a sense of responsibility. A comprehensive review of the patient can be achieved through the use of the care plan. The student who has cared for a patient is in the best position to evaluate and report on his or her progress. Although a monologue from the ward sister may take less time, the full potential of the ward report for teaching is not reached. A good report will also contribute to improved care of the patient as well as the education of the learner.

Group sessions between senior staff and learners are also of value when ethical problems occur in the treatment of patients. Free discussion about attitudes to a problem will relieve anxiety, and mutual support can be obtained. Senior staff may have encountered a similar situation before and can contribute their experience to the discussion. The learner may view the problem from a new angle and introduce fresh ideas for consideration.

The use of new equipment can be demonstrated to a group of learners, as it would be time consuming to teach each student individually. Participation by the learners will stimulate questions and discussion. It is, however, essential that everyone can see the demonstration and hear what is being said. Therefore the size of the group must be limited. As there will be students of varying experience and ability, it is essential that the information is clearly presented to everyone while ensuring that the least able understand the demonstration. The teacher must also see that the interest of the more able student is maintained.

The learner should have the opportunity to participate in ward rounds and case conferences relating to patients in her care. Personnel other than ward staff will be involved, and the attention given to teaching learners may be small. The student can, however, learn much from listening to the exchange of views, and can contribute by reporting her own observation of the patient.

The content of informal discussions will be unpredictable and cover a wide variety of material. Within the ward learning programme, it will also be necessary to plan structured tutorials when set subjects are discussed.

Tutorials

Tutorials should be arranged during a ward allocation so that the learner covers specific subjects relevant to her clinical experience. These tutorials can take many different forms, but all should relate to patient care. The session may cover the background anatomy and physiology necessary for the understanding of diseases treated on the ward. The implications for the nursing care of a patient with specific disease can be discussed in full.

The learner may present a history of one of the patients to illustrate particular points about treatment and care. Tutorial time may be allocated to a discussion of ethical problems, or to a general talk about ward policy. The leader of the tutorial can be anyone involved in patient care, and the group may sometimes include the patient.

The tutorials must be relevant and stimulating. As they usually occur in the afternoon, the learners may be tired and sleepy after a busy morning and a big lunch. Concentration will be further impaired if the accommodation is poor and there are constant interruptions from telephone calls or enquiries. A suitable place for ward tutorials is often hard to find as they must be held near the ward. A sudden emergency in the ward would necessitate extra staff and thus signal the end of the teaching session. Facilities should be available for presenting visual aids which will help to maintain interest.

The tutorials must cater for learners of differing abilities and experience. Students with more knowledge of a subject should be involved in teaching the others in the group. As junior students may feel reluctant to ask questions, material must be presented clearly to facilitate understanding. All learners should be encouraged to participate in the sessions.

Tutorials are an essential part of ward learning, and they and the other methods of teaching must be drawn together in the formulation of the ward learning programme.

The ward learning programme

When the ward learning programme is being planned, the needs of the learners and those of the ward must be balanced to achieve maximum benefit for both. It is pointless allocating hours of teaching to irrelevant material. Yet it is also unrealistic to expect one hour of teaching time per week to be sufficient to cover the information required for good patient care.

Decisions should be made at the outset on what is to be covered in the programme. Its content will obviously be considered in relation to the ward learning objectives. The specialist experience available on the ward will indicate areas for teaching. Note should be made of particular skills and types of care not practised elsewhere. The subjects should be relevant to the needs of the students at all stages of training. It must always be kept in mind that the nurse cannot be expected to become an expert in the speciality from a short allocation.

The ward staff should discuss the reasons behind the introduction of the learning programme. If they are not motivated to implement the programme it will not run effectively. The expected benefits of improved knowledge and nursing care by the learner can be summarised in aims and objectives. These will be stated in general terms for the whole allocation. For example, it can be stated that 'By the end of the ward allocation the student will be able to catheterise a female patient, using an aseptic and atraumatic technique', or 'By the end of the ward allocation the student will be able to identify five potential problems associated with catheterization'. These guidelines for learning should be given to the student at the beginning of her time on the ward. More precise objectives for individual teaching and tutorials should also be listed. These are of particular value when a student misses a session. She is then able to cover the same ground, using the objectives set by the ward.

The length of the whole learning programme must be determined. If students are allocated to the ward for eight-week periods, it is sensible to have a rotating cycle of an eight-week programme. The content of the programme should follow a logical sequence. In practice, the student will necessarily miss some continuity because of days off and night duty. Also, learners will commence their ward allocations at different points in the eight-week cycle. A programme planned on a weekly module, plus the provision of learning objectives, will provide the most successful answer to these problems.

The time in the week the sessions take place depends on the demands of the ward and on the availability of teachers. The afternoon may be the best time, as the patients are resting and having visitors. Also in many hospitals there is an overlap of nursing staff in the afternoon. It is, however, unrealistic to plan a teaching session for a busy day when operations and doctors' rounds are in full swing. The number of teaching sessions, and the time allotted to each, must be realistically planned, the demands of the ward being matched with the need to provide teaching opportunities. Once this is decided, off-duty may need to be adjusted to allow for the teaching commitment.

As mentioned earlier, a suitable 'classroom' must be found near the ward where teaching can take place and visual aids can be presented. This will not always be used as visits to departments or ward rounds may form part of the programme.

Discussion about how each subject is to be covered will identify who is needed to do the teaching. A variety of people will be involved and should be brought into the planning of the programme. The teaching method to be used must also be decided. Revision of aseptic technique may best be covered by one-to-one teaching, whereas the care of the terminally ill patient may best be discussed at a tutorial.

All this information can be drawn together and an appropriate ward learning timetable formulated (Table 3.2). The programme

Table 3.2. Ward learning programme – gynaeconogy experience. Time Table of forman sessions.

Week	Monday	Tuesday	Wednesday	Thursday	Friday	Saturday	Sunday
1.	Current trends in gynaecology	Teaching / report or ward round		Revision of relevant anatomy and physiology	/	Pre-operative care planning	Student project – case study
2.	Total patient care in gynaecology	Teaching report or ward round		Revision of menstrual cycle/ sex hormones	/	Post-operative care planning	Student project – case study
3.	Assessment of common gynaecological problems	Teaching / report or ward round		Investigation of gynaecological problems	/	Gynaecology nursing skills	Student project – case study
4.	Care plan – prolapse & repair	Teaching / report or ward round		Infections of genital tract/ ectopic pregnancy	/	Catheter-isation	Student project – case study
5.	Care plan – hysterectomy	Teaching report or ward round		Needs of patient with malignant disease	/	Emergency care	/Student project – case study
6.	Care plan – 'infertility'	Teaching / report or ward round		Hormonal treatment and drugs in gynaecology	/	Involving the family in care	Student project – case study
7.	Abortion	Teaching / report or ward round		Abortion – seminar	/	Nursing care wounds and drains	Student project – case study
8.	Genetic counselling	Teaching / report or ward round		Research in gynaecological nursing	/	Contra-ception	Student project – case study
	Clinical teacher	Ward staff or doctor		Tutor/ specialist staff		Ward staff	Learner

must be available for the student to see at the beginning of her allocation. Preparation for the sessions and follow-up reading are then the responsibility of the student.

A workbook of worksheets can be produced by the ward staff to complement the ward learning programme (Table 3.3).

Table 3.3 Worksheet – gynaecology experience

Prolapses and repairs

For the next section it would be useful to revise the anatomy of the pelvis, with particular reference to the muscles and ligaments.

1. What do you understand by the following terms:
   a. Cystocele
   b. Urethrocele
   c. Enterocele
   d. Procidentia
   e. Stress incontinence

2. What predisposing factors may lead to uterine prolapse?

3. Show by simple diagrams the three stages of uterine prolapse.

4. Describe the main methods used to treat a uterine prolapse.

5. List the possible presenting problem/needs of a patient with a cystocele.

6. What is done in the following operations?
   a. Posterior Colpoperineorrhaphy
   b. Marshall Marchetti
   c. Manchester Repair
   d. Vaginal Hysterectomy

7. Outline, in the form of a problem-orientated care plan, the post-operative care of one patient you have nursed following an anterior colporrhaphy.

8. What advice is given to a patient on discharge from hospital who has undergone either a hysterectomy or repair surgery?

The workbook given to each student at the start of the allocation will provide further guidelines for learning. The information required to complete the 'book' should all be available from the ward resources. The worksheets should also provide pointers for further study and information about relevant research. At the end of the allocation, the student and ward sister can review the completed workbook and the student can evaluate the effectiveness of the programme. Constant review and revision of the learning programme must be undertaken to ensure its continuing relevance.

Every ward should be considered a learning resource centre for each speciality, with the ward sister, in effect, the librarian. By the development of the ward programme, the full potential of the resource will be realized; but to plan an effective programme, the ward sister and staff need to be aware of the advantages and problems of bedside learning. They have at their disposal a wide variety of teaching methods and of teachers. The learner is allocated to the ward for such a short period that every learning opportunity must be exploited to the full. The onus, however, is on the student to obtain full benefit from the programme initiated by the ward staff. The student must not be allowed to leave the ward with the feeling expressed by Sir John Davies in *Nosce Teipsum*:

'Skill comes so slow, and life so fast doth fly,
We learn so little and forget so much.'

Summary

The aim of this chapter has been to discuss the opportunities and problems associated with ward learning. These are related specifically to the personnel involved in ward teaching and the methods by which the teaching is undertaken. The responsibility of the student to take opportunities for learning has been stressed. Finally, suggestions have been made for improving ward learning by the introduction of a planned programme. This includes teaching sessions, and the use of worksheets and all other learning resources available in the ward. For the success of ward learning, evaluation of both the ward programme and the progress of the student is vital.

REFERENCES

Allen, H.O. (1982) *The Ward Sister: Role and Preparation*. London: Bailliere Tindall.

Bendall, E. (1975) *So You Passed, Nurse*. London: Royal College of Nursing.

Fretwell, J. E. (1980) An inquiry into the ward learning environment. Occasional Papers, *Nursing Times*, 76(16), 69–75.

Fretwell, J. E. (1982) *Ward Teaching and Learning*. London: Royal College of Nursing. 76.

H.M.S.O. London (1972) Command No. 5115 Report of the Committee on Nursing (Chairman – Professor Asa Briggs).

Lewis, D.C. & Leach, J. (1983) Factors influencing the quality of wards as learning environments for student nurses. *International Journal of Nursing Studies*, 19(3), 125–137.

Ogier, M. E. (1982) (1982) IAn Ideal Sister? London: Royal College of Nursing.

Orton, H.D. (1981) *Ward Learning Climate*. London: Royal College of Nursing.

Pembrey, S. (1980) *The Ward Sister – Key to Nursing*. London: Royal College of Nursing.

Stockwell, F. (1972) *The Unpopular Patient*. London: Royal College of Nursing.

Weed, L.L. (1969) *Medical Records: Medical Education and Patient Care*. Cleveland Press of Case Western Reserve University.

FURTHER READING

Roper, N. (1976) *Clinical Experience in Nurse Education*. University of Edinburgh, Department of Nursing Studies. Monograph No. 5. Edinburgh: Churchill Livingstone.

Sheahen, J. (1976) Education – teaching skills and teaching aids. *Nursing Times*, Steptember 30, pp 1526–1528. Communication Skills and Assessment Learning. *Nursing Times*, October 7, pp 1570–1572.

4

Aims and objectives

The purpose of teaching is to bring about changes in students through the medium of planned experiences. Statements describing proposed changes are normally referred to as aims and objectives. In this chapter, we shall examine the nature of these two concepts and estimate their value for teachers.

Although these terms are sometimes used interchangeably, it is useful to distinguish between them. An aim can be taken to be a statement of intent on the part of the teacher, usually expressed in general terms, whilst an objective is a statement describing in specific terms what the student is expected to do at the end of a course of learning experience.

Consider the following:

1. To introduce the students to the practice of nursing.
2. To provide an introduction to basic physiology.
3. To develop an understanding of the psychological aspects of nursing care.
4. To develop an understanding of the principles of therapeutic diets.
5. To introduce the postoperative medical and nursing care of patients with peripheral vascular disease.
6. To extend the student's understanding of psychiatric conditions, their treatment and nursing care.
7. To provide practical experience of the nursing care of patients with respiratory disorders.

These are aims and could be prefixed by the statement 'The teacher intends . . . .' They are general in nature in that they indicate broad areas of content and could be achieved in a variety of ways. Aims are necessary starting points, but before the teacher can begin to provide learning experiences further refinement is necessary. How, for example, is one to know that the students have an understanding of therapeutic diets? Which diets are involved? Are these to be learned all at once and how are they best learned? How is the teacher to tell that her teaching has been successful? These and many other questions will need answers before teaching can begin. The first step is to translate aims into objectives, that is to state exactly what is expected of the students.

Compare the following list of objectives with the above aims:

The student will be able to:

1. Make up a bed according to standard procedure, for a post-operative thyroidectomy patient.
2. Prepare a day's diet sheet for a Gujurati Hindu patient with chronic renal failure, taking into account relevant medical and religious constraints.
3. Given a particular post-operative patient in the recovery phase, draw up and execute a plan of nursing care for the first twenty-four hours.

It will be seen at once that these statements are more specific and precise than aims, which raises an important question. What degree of precision is necessary? Objective (1) could be written in more detail. We could specify in which hand the draw-sheet is to be held, which arm the nurse is to use to support the patient, the degree of tension to be applied to the draw-sheet to make it taut and smooth. We could specify what words the student will say to the patient and even at what point she is to smile. There is, in fact, no single answer to this question. The degree of precision in objectives will depend on the intentions of the teacher, the experience of the student and the nature of the activities involved. If the teacher's intention is to give a general overview or introduction to a topic, then less detail will be needed. Where students are already experienced then perhaps some very precise detail will be required. Some nursing skills require a higher degree of precision than others: compare, for example, the post-operative care of a patient carrying the sickle cell trait with that of one who does not, or bed-making for patients in traction and for more active patients.

Objectives, then, should reflect the teacher's intentions and should be appropriate for the students and for the activity involved. On the whole this is a matter of the teacher exercising her professional judgement both as a nurse and a teacher, but there are a variety of ideas available to help her in devising objectives. Some of these we will consider next.

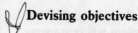

Devising objectives

Three useful conditions have been advocated by which a teacher may judge her objectives. These are:

1. That objectives should be unambiguous.
2. That they should specify the conditions under which the final behaviour will occur.
3. That they should indicate the standard to be reached.

We shall deal with each one in turn. Ambiguity can arise from two sources:

1. Lack of clarity on the part of the teacher about the task being taught.
2. Lack of clarity about the outcome or final performance required.

Clarity about the nature of the task involved can be achieved by carrying out a task analysis. This consists of breaking down the task into its constituent parts and compiling a list of the skills and knowledge involved, thus composing a recipe for the successful performance of the task. Where practical skills are involved, this may take the form of observing someone perform the task (a competent nurse in this case) and recording in detail what she actually does.

At first glance this may seem a tedious and unnecessary task, for any nurse aspiring to teach others ought to be sufficiently proficient at nursing not to require this kind of reminder. However, the matter is not so simple. Nurses who have been nursing for some time are likely to have reached the stage where much of what they do has become automatic, that is, carried out without conscious thought or awareness. It is quite easy when teaching a novice, especially in the earlier stages of teaching, to omit important details and to omit explanations and justifications for what is done. These are often vital for a beginner, because they give meaning to the tasks involved. Some form of task analysis is necessary therefore, either in the form of observation or introspective reconstruction, in order to write unambiguous objectives.

The second source of ambiguity, confusion about the final performance required, is slightly different from the above source and is perhaps more common in teaching. It occurs when teaching programmes do not relate to the final assessment of learning. A common example is the situation in which students find themselves being asked questions on topics that have not been taught. A less obvious and regrettably a more common example is where students are presented throughout the course with bodies of facts and procedures to be remembered and applied as faithfully as possible; then in the final testing they are assessed on their ability to apply their knowledge and skills to new situations, or to explain, justify and discuss the reasons behind procedures. Now all of these require more complex intellectual abilities than simple remembering, and therefore need to be included in the teaching programme and reflected in the form the objectives take. This illustrates the important link between objectives and assessment. Ambiguity, then, can be avoided by having a clear understanding of the abilities and capabilities that are going to be assessed. This will be reflected in the choice of words used in objectives. It will be noted that these begin with a verb stating the actions students are expected to show. Some verbs are more ambiguous than others. Consider the following two lists:

(a)	(b)
understand	describe
know	list
grasp the meaning of	prepare
appreciate	demonstrate
show an interest in	contrast
acquire	state.

The meanings of the words in list (a) are not as clear as those in list (b). How does one know that someone 'understands' or 'knows' something? One can only tell by asking the person to do something such as 'state' or 'demonstrate'. Clarity in objectives can be achieved by using the latter terms. A simple test for ambiguity in the two lists can be made by asking a number of people to say, separately, what they would expect to see, if they were asked to mark students showing the capabilities given in the two lists. Close agreement indicates some degree of precision, whilst general disagreement about a word suggests that it is ambiguous.

One important difference between the two lists is that those in list (a) refer to internal events and states, whilst those in list (b) denote external and therefore observable behaviour. Words such as those in list (b) are more suitable for writing objectives. Of course, we want our students to know, understand and appreciate the things we are teaching, but these terms represent our intentions and are more suitably expressed as aims. The simple test for ambiguity in an objective is to ask the question: Does this objective state what the nurse is going to do to show me that she has learned? This, then is the first condition for successful objectives – lack of ambiguity.

The second condition is that it must specify the conditions under which the behaviour will occur. This consists of including a statement of those things with which the nurse is to be provided in order to demonstrate her final level of performance. In our three examples of objectives given above, these conditions are specified. In (1) we are not asking the student to make up any bed but a particular kind of bed for a particular patient. The conditions are laid down. Similarly, 'for a Gujurati Hindu with chronic renal failure,' and 'given a post-operative patient in the recovery phase' specify different conditions and limits. In the latter case, the nurse is free to choose which post-operative condition she is to work on. What limits a teacher wishes to set will depend entirely on her own intentions for a given student. A different kind of limitation is set by the third condition and it is this which we will look at now.

The third requirement (that an objective should indicate the standard to be reached) is probably the most difficult one to meet, for it embraces a whole range of problems and issues that are perhaps best dealt with under the heading of assessment. Nevertheless it is not something that we can ignore, for the teacher needs feedback from her students' performances in order to judge the effectiveness of her teaching and may need to know that students have reached certain standards before progressing to more difficult work. Students also need to know what standards are required of them. All too often they have to guess what is in the minds of their teachers. Those who make the right guesses early on are often seen as 'good' or intelligent students; those who do not are often labelled slow or stupid.

The problem lies in determining what the standards shall be. In some cases they are provided: making up a two per cent solution means two per cent not one per cent or ten, giving ten millilitres of medication is a precise measure, but it is not always so easy to define standards.

Sometimes there are 'standard' requirements to be met. These may be standard to nursing in general, or locally determined. Institutions often have their own expectations, and provided all are agreed within an institution the teacher may draw on them. It is this kind of situation that is indicated in the first objective in the examples above. For example, the objective 'make up a bed, according to standard procedure' draws on general standards in that waterproof pillow-covers and light bedding would be required, and local standards for bed making, whether that means a 'general tucking-in all round' or 'all corners perfectly rectangular and with the top sheet turned over 32.5 cms'.

This appeal to local standards does not solve the problems, but merely moves the solution from the shoulders of teachers, which may or may not be a good thing. The important point for the teacher to remember is that local agreement about standards does not in any sense make them absolute. In some nursing situations, establishing criteria for objective assessment involves procedures that are too technically complicated or too time consuming to be attempted. Judgements of students are often made on the basis of the subjective values of teachers or ward staff, that is, on what is believed to be good practice. This seems to apply particularly in the area of nurse – patient relationships. It is commonly accepted that part of a nurse's functions is to be sensitive to and provide care for the psychological needs of patients, achieved in part through interpersonal relationships. If students are to be assessed on this aspect of their performance, it ought to be included in any teaching programme and in the teacher's objectives. The difficulty is not so much in defining the content for a given situation as stating the level of performance required. If this is doubted, try to write a set of objectives, including criteria for assessment, for the psychological care of an elderly middle class lady who has just had a colostomy performed. It is not that these judgements should not be made, but that where subjective judgements are made by the teacher she should be aware that this is so and be prepared, not only to give reasons for her judgements, but also to be sufficiently flexible to change them in the light of particular circumstances.

There are three further points to be made about writing objectives. The first is that it is usually preferable to make each objective refer to only one learning outcome. Example (3) falls down in this respect in that it includes two different activities and outcomes: 'to draw up a plan', and 'to execute it'. If both of these activities are to be taught, then two objectives are needed so that we can distinguish between failures of planning and failures in execution. If the student is known to be competent at planning, and it is the details of execution we are to teach, then a double objective would be acceptable.

The second point is that the writing of objectives has a purpose. It enables teachers to make clear statements about what they want their students to do, but it is not always necessary or possible to satisfy all of the conditions given above. Considerable variations in format are possible, depending on what the teacher wants her students to achieve as a result of her teaching.

Finally, the purpose of this section has been to help teachers write clear objectives. Whether or not the content and outcomes in nursing or educational terms are worthwhile is an entirely different matter. One could write clear, concise objectives for a completely irrelevant content, and one's teaching of it could be improved, but this would in no way justify the use of an irrelevant curriculum. Objectives form part of the technology of the teaching process.

In order to appreciate the value of objectives, it is useful to examine the part they can play in the teaching process. There is a variety of models for teaching, perhaps as many as there are

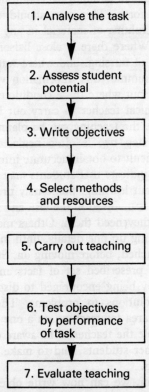

Fig. 4.1   A systems model for teaching

teachers, but the one that provides the most logical context for objectives is the systems model illustrated in diagrammatic form in Figure 4.1. In this model the planning and teaching process is analysed into a sequence of logical steps. It begins after the aims and general content for a period of ward experience have been defined. Once the task to be taught has been selected we can begin the first step in the model, that of analysing the task into its component elements and plotting the knowledge and skills necessary for successful performance. Not only does this provide us with the content to be taught, but it also lays the foundation on which final assessment can be based; however, before we can devise our objectives, two further collections of information are needed. These are obtained by step two. Here we check to ensure that the students have the knowledge and skills necessary to begin the piece of learning. This may include knowledge of technical terms and procedures, background knowledge of relevant anatomy and physiology, knowledge of pathological conditions, related signs and symptoms and so forth. This step should ensure that the difficulty level and the volume of material in any one session are right for the students. Where there is close liaison between ward teachers and the school of nursing, and where ward experience is part of a planned programme, this information will be available from previous teaching; but where these conditions do not exist it is necessary for the clinical teacher to carry out her own checks with the students before the teaching can be planned.

The second part of step two is often neglected by teachers, mainly because it is difficult to obtain accurate information. There is sufficient evidence to indicate that students may differ markedly in the ways they set about learning. Some may prefer to be given a global picture of what is involved in the task and then be allowed to fill in the details as they need them. Others may prefer a step by step process of building up fine details, until mastery of a sub-section of the task is reached, before moving on. Some may prefer to be presented with a prescribed set of facts and skills, whilst others may learn best by being encouraged to discover things for themselves, often as solutions to problems. The opportunities provided in the clinical area for teaching on a one to one or small group basis should enable the teacher to be aware of at least some of these differences in her students, and to make some provision for them in her teaching.

Using this information, we can now write objectives that will achieve that stated aims and will be appropriate for the task and the students' differences and needs. They will also form the basis for assessment in step six.

The selection of methods and resources is a major topic in itself, for just as there is no one best method of learning there is no one best method of teaching. The main criterion is that the methods selected should be the best available for achieving the selected objectives for a known group of students. However the realities of the clinical area impose constraints on both methods and resources, so that in achieving a satisfactory compromise between the ideal and what is possible the teacher may find her imagination and ingenuity tested to the full.

A second constraint, one that is often overlooked, comes from the teacher herself. Just as students differ in preferred methods of learning, so do teachers differ in preferred methods of teaching. The bases of these differences seem to be not only differences in acquired knowledge and skills, but also in intellectual and person- ality characteristics, that is in styles of thinking and styles of social interaction. Competence in teaching means having sufficient insight into the teacher's own weaknesses, strengths and preferences to enable her to adapt her methods so that she is comfortable in using them.

We now have three criteria for the selection of methods and resources: that they should be appropriate for the objectives and the students to be taught; that they should be practicable in the context of the teaching session; and that they should be compatible with the personal resources of the teacher.

Once the teaching has been carried out, it remains to test formally or informally that the objectives have been achieved. In this model, testing consists of checking that the students can carry out the task by the criteria detailed in the objectives. It is here that the value of well thought-out objectives can be seen. All too often teachers intend to teach one thing, actually teach another, and test for something quite different. As objectives are translations of intentions into statements of final competence, this confusion is less likely to happen. In cases where students achieve all objectives satisfactorily, step six provides information for step two of the next related teaching programme.

The final step provides an evaluation or post-mortem of the whole teaching programme so that, in cases where students have not achieved the objectives, appropriately modified plans can be made for future teaching. This process of continuous evaluation, if carried out conscientiously, will lead to more effective teaching.

The systematic model of teaching illustrates how influential correctly used objectives can be on the whole teaching process from planning to assessment, and demonstrates the need for extreme care in choosing them. We can turn now to a closer examination of the kinds of objectives possible.

There is a tendency when first writing objectives to limit them to simple forms of behaviour, such as the reproduction of facts and the demonstration of skills; but if we, as teachers, are to offer our students anything more than simple training, we must be able to devise objectives that describe more complex operations.

One model that provides a basis for objectives is the Taxonomy of Educational Objectives, published by Bloom and his associates (Bloom, B. S. *et al.*, 1956). In this model, educational goals are divided into three fields or domains, each representing a different aspect of human functioning.

The domains are:
1. Cognitive: embracing the intellectual abilities of remembering, conceptualisation and reasoning.
2. Affective: emphasising the emotional qualities of feelings, attitudes, interests and values.
3. Psychomotor: emphasising the development of motor skills.

Each domain is subdivided into a hierarchy of categories, which provide the basis for a set of objectives for a given piece of learning.

In the cognitive domain (Table 4.1), the categories are: knowledge, comprehension, application, analysis, synthesis and evaluation. They are arranged in order of increasing complexity. Table 4.1 presents the categories with the abilities that teachers could aim to develop in column one and in column two some terms for use in corresponding objectives.

The following is an example of some cognitive objectives for teaching the nursing care of a patient recovering from heart surgery.

The student will be able to:
1. Describe the nursing interventions prescribed (knowledge)
2. Give reasons for each step (comprehension)
3. Carry out the care for a given patient (application)
4. State the underlying principles for post-operative care of a patient following heart surgery (analysis)
5. Plan and execute the post-operative care for a second patient (different condition) (synthesis)

Table 4.1 The cognitive domain

Cognitive categories	Terms used in objectives
Knowledge Student knows common terms, facts, concepts, methods and procedures.	Define, identify, state, describe.
Comprehension Understands facts, interprets, charts graphs, predicts consequences.	Explain, give new examples of, infer, predict.
Application Uses material in new situation, applies theory to practice.	Demonstrate, solve new problems, use in new situation, apply in practice.
Analysis Understands the organisational principles and structures in the material.	Identify principles, relate, distinguish between.
Synthesis Compiles new procedures and plans from above knowledge.	Devise nursing care plan, organise, work for, create.
Evaluation Judges value of material and procedures, either on the basis of the material or the end results.	Appraise, compare one method of care with another, explain, justify.

6. Evaluate the effectiveness of the plan for satisfying the medical, psychological, and personal needs of the patients and for catering for potential problems. (evaluation).

In practice a set of objectives like these would be written for a series of teaching sessions for a specific student or group and may be varied to suit their experience and needs. Objectives (1) and (2) could consist of checks after a preliminary period of revision or practice carried out by the student on her own. The teaching and practice sessions for objective (3) may consists of several guided experiences with different patients, for which subsidiary objectives may be needed. The teaching for objectives (3) and (5) may, in practice, run together as increasing competence enables the nurse to take more responsibility for the work.

The affective domain is similarly divided into a hierarchy of five categories. These are: receiving, responding, valuing, organisation, characterisation by value complex. Table 4.2 gives the main interpretations of each category and some terms for related objectives. The first two categories represent the initial stages of involvement in learning to be a nurse. The final three categories represent the progressive development of a professional style of nursing, in which patterns of personal, social and emotional functioning in all aspects of the work are sufficiently self-disciplined to enable the nurse to work effectively. The nurse should strive for the middle way between total involvement in the job dominating her personal life to the point where her development as a person is impaired and her health jeopardised; and the other extreme in which she may be technically proficient, but appears totally detached from the work both emotionally and socially. In this model this desirable 'professional style' consists of collections or sets of values attached to different aspects of the work (such as the administration of drugs, carrying out aseptic technique, basic theoretical knowledge such as anatomy, physiology, pathology and so on), organised into a complex structure which characterises the nurse's attitudes to the work.

Table 4.2 The affective domain

Categories: affective domain	Terms used in objectives
Receiving Student listens, shows sensitivity to human needs, attends closely to teaching.	Ask questions, follow, respond to questions from teacher or patient.
Responding Student actively participates in learning.	Discuss, help, perform, report on.
Valuing Student behaviour reflects internalised set of values.	Initiate, justify
Organisation of values Student brings together different sets of values; shows internal consistency.	Defend, compare, explain, order, organise, prepare.
Characterisation by values Value system controls student's behaviour, so that she is consistent in a wide variety of situations.	Act consistently, influence, verify.

It seems difficult to write behavioural objectives for this domain alone, as affective functioning is always interwoven with cognitive functioning. In the examples of objectives given above for the cognitive domain, the affective component will be revealed in the quality of the interaction between the student and patient, in the way the nurse handles any complications arising, and in the evaluation stage, in the emphasis she places on personal and psychological needs.

It may be argued that because the affective domain deals with qualitative differences it cannot be planned for in the same systematic way that is applied to knowledge, and that it is best dealt with by providing suitable models, and by discussion when problems and student needs arise. It may also be argued that, as this field is concerned with aspects of the student that are intimately connected with her personality, it would be unethical to attempt systematically to bring about changes. This could be seen as indoctrination and not education.

The motor skills domain has received far less attention than the cognitive and affective, and objectives in this field are perhaps best devised from a study of the way skills are learned. The principles described above still apply in that skills are especially suited to analysis, and can be assessed more easily than the other domains by objective tests.

Evaluation of aims and objectives

We can now turn to assessing the value of these ideas for education in general and clinical teaching in particular. There can be little doubt about the need for the clear formal statement of the aims of nurse education. Teaching is a purposive activity, so that even though the teacher or school may not formulate aims consciously they will be implicit in the teaching, and will influence the course of the student's education. As the purpose of teaching is to produce a planned change in students, it is essential that those whose responsibility it is to produce the change should be clear not only about their intentions but about the assumptions on which those intentions are based. The process of formally stating aims can be instrumental in bringing about an examination of assumptions if undertaken in a self-searching way. Translating aims into specific objectives can assist in removing the confusions that can arise between intentions and practice, but beyond this the case for objectives is less certain; in fact, it has been one of the most hotly debated innovations in teaching for some time. For a comprehensive review of this debate the relevant chapters in Stenhouse (1975) are recommended. The advantages and disadvantages of objectives can be examined from several viewpoints but we will confine ourselves to three: the practical, ethical and educational.

From the practical standpoint, it is often claimed that there is never enough time to write objectives; that their use removes the spontaneity from teaching; and finally that from a clinical point of view they are inappropriate, as much of the teaching is 'crisis' teaching and cannot be foreseen nor planned.

The question of time can be answered in two ways. Teachers become more efficient at writing objectives the more they practise, so that they can soon reach the stage where the time taken is no more than is required for planning anyway. Of course one needs to exercise some common sense about the number of objectives written for any one piece of teaching, but if teaching sessions are seen as part of a series for a given student then objectives can be written for the whole series. This seems the most appropriate way to use Bloom's *Taxonomy* (1956) in clinical teaching.

Objections on the grounds of time often disguise a more fundamental problem which concerns teaching in general and not just the objectives model. It is reasonably accurate to say that good teaching comes largely from thorough planning, yet all too often far too little planning time is made available. Where this is the case, it is the teacher's responsibility to present the best case she can for more time to those who devise her timetable. She must also become more efficient herself in the use of the time available. Formal planning strategies can assist in this.

Loss of spontaneity is a different kind of criticism. It is true that occasionally experienced teachers can give good, seemingly spontaneous, teaching. This is usually due less to some brilliant inspiration of the moment than to a skilful adaptation of previously made and polished plans and techniques, and is therefore a product of planning rather than an alternative to it. Brilliant, spontaneous teaching is a rare event, and it would be a disservice to students to abandon planning in the hope that such teaching might happen.

The question of crisis teaching needs closer examination. We need to know what a teacher can do in a crisis that could be called teaching. It seems that the teacher cannot do much more than demonstrate applied knowledge and nursing skills, applied personal resources, and the skills required in modifying and adapting a variety of procedures to meet particular contingencies. A demonstration is only part of the teaching process; the rest, such as the presentation and analysis of the theoretical knowledge on which the procedures are based, the teaching and practice of necessary skills, the evaluation of the procedures, and extension work such as the construction of contingency plans for related but different emergencies, must take place in follow-up sessions. If this is not done then the teaching and learning are left unfinished. Follow-up sessions can be planned and suitable objectives devised for the student. In this way the unplanned crisis serves as a powerful stimulus for further, planned teaching and therefore does not preclude the use of objectives.

A stronger criticism of the use of objectives can be made on ethical grounds. This view argues that it is undemocratic and unethical to change deliberately another person's behaviour. This is usually countered by arguing that there is a basic selection of knowledge and skills that a nurse must have to ensure competence, and teachers and curriculum planners are in a better position than students to know what these are. Secondly, the student volunteers to become a nurse and therefore consents to being guided by those who know what is required. Whilst there is some truth in both of these arguments, they are open to question. The superior knowledge of the teacher does not automatically invest her with the right to place students in an intellectual straitjacket, nor does volunteering to be a nurse mean that one has automatically signed away one's rights as a human being. The real point at issue here is not *whether* objectives should be used but *how* they are used. They can become a rigid system for controlling students and teachers, but they need not be used in this way. If objectives from the higher categories of Bloom's taxonomy are included, where students are asked to make judgements, to criticise and evaluate; and if students are given a range of objectives from which they may make their own choices and even, at the later stages of training, are encouraged to write their own, then this will go a long way to meeting this criticism.

The most fundamental criticism raised on educational grounds is that objectives may be suitable for training programmes but are not suitable for education. The heart of the matter is the distinction made between these two concepts. Training is seen as the acquisition of knowledge and skills for a specific purpose. The trained person applies them in ways that are laid down during training. Education is seen to include some of this, but goes a long way beyond competence in application. It stimulates the development of rational thinking, of critical and creative abilities so that an educated person is able to employ any knowledge and skills she may have in a variety of ways and contexts. The concern is more with the development of the student's mind, not solely with behaviour. There is no simple formula by which this may be achieved, and its very nature makes it impossible to draw up a catalogue of final behaviours to be acquired. The educated person is characterised less by what she can do, and more by what the process of learning and knowing has done to her.

There is no easy soution to the education versus training argument in nursing. If the clinical teacher sees her role as a trainer developing competence then objectives can be applied; but if she sees herself as providing something more than this, perhaps aiding and encouraging the development of the nurse as an autonomous person within the context of nursing, then she will go beyond the stage where objectives can be applied.

This criticism is sometimes expressed in another way. The question often raised is 'should education be so dominated by assessment?' Many teachers argue that the more important things that they are concerned with, the 'something more', are qualities that cannot be measured by tests of competence; if teaching is geared to what can be measured, objectives in other words, then these important qualities will be omitted and both the teaching and students will be the poorer. Where a teacher feels this is likely to happen it becomes her responsibility to see that the danger is avoided.

Where objectives are used appropriately the model does have some advantages. One advantage is that the students are not in competition with each other, as each student's achievement is assessed against the criteria laid down and not against the best student. Given time, it is theoretically possible for all students to gain 100 per cent marks.

Two further advantages are that objectives provide the student with a clear idea of what is expected of her and that teachers are forced to think clearly about what they expect of students.

The best conclusion that one can draw is that the objectives model provides a useful tool for certain purposes, especially the basic levels of knowledge and skill acquisition, but that is should not be used exclusively nor without judgement.

REFERENCES

Bloom, B. S. et. al. (1956) Taxonomy of Educational Objectives. I. Cognitive Domain. London: Longman.
Krathwohl, D. R. et. al. (1964) Taxonomy of Educational Objectives. II. Affective Domain. London: Longman.
Stenhouse, L. (1975) An Introduction to Curriculum Research and Development. London: Heinemann.
Mager, R. F. (1962) Preparing Instructional Objectives. Palo Alto: Fearon.

5

Approaches to learning

Almost everything we do in our daily lives whether it be driving a car, making tea, or solving complex professional problems on the ward, is directly or indirectly the result of learning. It is not surprising, therefore, to find that learning has been one of the most extensively studied of human abilities, yet we do not have one complete explanatory theory that can guide teachers. A glance at any psychology textbook on the subject will reveal a variety of conflicting views about the nature and process of learning derived from widely different experiments with humans, rats, pigeons, monkeys, and even octopuses.

The reason for this diversity is that learning, like all mental processes, remains hidden. What takes place when someone learns something cannot be observed directly; we can only know that learning has taken place by examining changes in the person's behaviour after the event. Similarly we can only make inferences about the nature of learning from observing these changes. The problem is reflected in definitions of learning. The following are typical:

'Learning is a more or less permanent change in behaviour not due to maturation or damage.'
'Learning is a change in human disposition or capability which can be retained, and which is not simply ascribable to the process of growth.' *Gagné*

These definitions do not say what learning is, but describe it in terms of its effects.

One of the problems created by this hidden nature of learning is that it is not clear whether or not the same process is involved in widely different activities. Does learning to ride a bicycle or give an injection involve the same processes as learning the anatomy and physiology of the alimentary tract, or a foreign language, or learning to solve problems? At the beginning of this century it was

97

believed that one could find a basic element of learning that was common to all these activities; and that once this was established it would be possible to construct a single theory that would explain all learning and would provide a once-and-for-all guide to teaching. Several attempts were made to construct such a theory by such people as Watson, Thorndike, Hull, Tolman and Köhler and his colleagues. Eventually these theories fell into disuse, largely because they were unable to explain the whole range of different types of learning. Nevertheless, each theory contributed something to our understanding of the process.

In recent years it has become more acceptable to distinguish between different types of learning. Gagné (1970) – whose work we will examine later – has compiled a hierarchy of eight types, the purpose of which is to help the teacher to match her teaching to the kind of learning she wishes to produce.

When an experienced teacher is planning a learning experience, she asks herself at least three questions:

1. What is learning and which kind is involved in this activity?
2. What are the different conditions under which learning is most likely to take place?
3. What part can I play in bringing about this learning?

She may not formulate these questions consciously, but her planning and teaching will reflect the influence of these considerations. The purpose of this chapter is to examine some possible answers to these questions and to relate them to the clinical situation.

Types of learning

It is convenient to divide approaches to the study of learning into two broad categories:

1. Associative learning, which includes both classical and operant conditioning and emphasises mechanical connections or associations between events.
2. Cognition theories, which emphasise internal functions such as perception and understanding and see learning in terms of the organisation of mental connections which influence future performance.

Historically associative theories have their origins in the latter part of the last century in a reaction against current introspective approaches in psychology. This reaction produced attempts to apply scientific principles and procedures to the study of human functioning. Scientific method involves the precise measurement of observable events, which in the case of learning meant studying the measurable changes in behaviour. Principal workers in this field were Watson, Pavlov, Thorndike, Hull and the contemporary psychologist, Skinner.

The main concept in associative learning theory is that there is a basic unit of learning which consists of a more or less permanent connection between two events: a stimulus (S), which is any object or event that acts on an organism, and the reaction to it, or response (R) that the learner makes. Once the connection is made and established it is referred to as an S-R bond. The more frequently a response is paired with a particular stimulus, the more likely it is to become a permanent relationship or habit. Complex human behaviour is seen as established sequences or chains of S-R bonds. The teacher's function is to decide what these chains are to be and to take steps to establish them as permanent ways of responding.

Associative theories can be divided into two major fields, each offering a different way for establishing S-R bonds. These are classical and operant conditioning. We will deal briefly with these in turn, but for a fuller account the reader is recommended to Walker (1975).

In classical conditioning, learning consists of establishing a relationship between a natural response and a stimulus that would not normally evoke it. The basic experiment with dogs conducted by Pavlov (1925) will illustrate the principles.

Presented with food (S), dogs secrete saliva (R) before eating. This bond was referred to by Pavlov as 'unconditional' meaning innate and not dependent on previous learning.

Presented with the noise of a tuning fork, the dog will respond, by turning its head or cocking its ears, but will not salivate. The purpose of the experiment was to train the dog to salivate at the sound of the tuning fork without food being present. This was achieved by presenting the noise of the fork just before food was given, and then after some repetition presenting the noise of the fork alone.

Before training
1. Tuning fork (S)→Head turning
Training
2. Tuning fork plus food→Salivation (R)
After training
3. Tuning fork (S)→Salivation (R)

The dog had learned to associate the tuning fork with food and responded to it as though it were food. This new bond was called conditional (upon training) or conditioned. Two conditions are necessary for this kind of learning to occur. The first is called contiguity, which means that the two stimuli – the fork and the food – had to be presented simultaneously or at least close together. The second condition is that repetition or practice of this pairing was necessary.

Numerous experiments have been conducted involving different variations of the principles. Where Pavlov used pleasant stimuli, others have used unpleasant ones such as electric shocks. It has been found that this form of conditioning can occur much more rapidly if the response prevents unpleasant stimuli occurring or stops them once they have started. Eysenck, a contemporary British psychologist, has investigated classical conditioning with humans employing eye-blinking as the unconditional response. One important finding is that people differ in the number of repetitions needed to establish this kind of learning. The differences are thought to be functional differences in the nervous system. It seems that anxious people condition most easily and it is thought that irrational fears are established in this way.

As this is a very basic form of learning it is unlikely that the clinical teacher will find any direct applications of it in her teaching. One is more likely to see examples of the results of it however. Recovering patients rapidly acquire anticipatory responses to the noise of the tea trolley, and some patients may show excessive anxiety reactions to the sight of a hypodermic syringe. Perhaps more important for the teacher is that some students, especially those from other cultures, may have been conditioned to respond to authority figures, especially teachers, by unquestioning obedience. Such students may seem to lack initiative and may even be dismissed as dull. Working alongside the student as a nurse affords the clinical teacher opportunities to help such a student develop a more questioning attitude to nursing.

The second form of associative learning, operant conditioning, was developed by the contemporary American psychologist, Skinner, who not only conducted laboratory experiments with animals, but, unlike most other theorists, also developed from his findings teaching procedures for use with people, especially programmed learning and teaching machines.

The two necessary conditions of contiguity and repetition apply but the procedure is different. The basic principle in operant learning is that an item or sequence of behaviour is strengthened or weakened by its consequences. An operant is any item of behaviour shown by a person. If the behaviour brings about pleasant or rewarding consequences, it is more likely to be repeated. If on the other hand the consequences are neutral or unpleasant, then the behaviour is less likely to occur and an alternative will be found. Pleasant consequences are called reinforcers and the strengthening of the behaviour is called reinforcement.

Some variations of the basic model have been studied. If a reinforcer is given every time an operant is shown there is an initial rapid increase in the occurrence of that operant until a steady level of behaviour is reached. Once the reinforcer is stopped there is a decline in the rate of responding. If, on the other hand, the frequency of reinforcement is changed after the initial increase to an intermittent one, that is the person is rewarded only occasionally, then there is a further increase, and the behaviour is maintained long after the reinforcer is withdrawn. The learning has become more or less permanent. The technical term for intermittent reinforcement is 'partial reinforcement' and represents the most powerful way of developing and changing behaviour.

Selective reinforcement, the rewarding of required and approved behaviour, can be a useful technique for teachers, where praise and approval are used for shaping and maintaining desired student performance, especially in the early stages of learning when students need this kind of reassurance and when the work itself has not yet become intrinsically satisfying.

Associative learning provides explanations for basic forms of learning. It is unlikely, however, that a single S-R bond can be found in human learning, as most of the things we teach involve complex sequences or chains of responses. What this model suggests is that the acquisition of complex behaviour is analogous to constructing a wall, a process of building up a structure brick by brick. Whether or not this is acceptable depends on how one sees complex behaviour. Some would argue that such a view does not take into account the complex nature of the human mind. This opinion is held by those who advocate a cognitive approach to learning.

Cognition theories

Whereas associative theories emphasise the passive responding to external events and the building of complex behaviour from small elements, cognition theories emphasise the active engagement of the person and an organic model for the acquisition of complex behaviour. Between the presentation of stimuli and the responses made to them, a complex sequence of selecting, discriminating, organising and decision making is said to take place. The active engagement of the learner in this process has been studied extensively under the title perception. Successful nursing depends very largely on the nurse's ability to deal effectively with information received through the senses, whether it is obtained by formal means, such as taking blood-pressure, temperatures and so on or by informal means such as noticing changes in the patient's condition during bed-making. Some information is registered and acted upon, other information may register but be stored and recalled later whilst other information may not be registered at all. There seems general agreement that the mind does not work like a camera, faithfully recording everything in front of its lens, for apart from the discrimination of sensations and the filtering out of some of them, the information that is passed on undergoes considerable re-organisation and change so that there is always a discrepancy between the sensory input and what is perceived. It is on these final percepts that judgements and consequent action are based. Formal observation techniques and equipment are designed to reduce this discrepancy to a minimum but the nursing process depends on much more than can be obtained by this means; therefore it is important for the teacher to have some understanding of the factors that affect the formation of percepts so that she can help the nurse to make accurate judgements where these are possible and to be sufficiently receptive and mentally flexible to consider more than one possible judgement as basis for action. This understanding is important for teaching too, because whatever the teacher intends the student to learn, she will learn her own approximations to it.

A variety of factors in the stimuli presented have been found to influence selection. Intense, novel and variable stimuli are attended to rather than others, whilst regularly repeated stimuli seem to become ignored. The organisation of material once it has been attended to was extensively studied by Gestalt psychologists. Their basic proposition was that we tend to organise and simplify incoming information until it makes a satisfying pattern. Similar information tends to be grouped together, whilst missing information tends to be completed from what is available, or from experience. The value for teachers of this information is that, by

presenting the content of their teaching in a pattern that is satisfying to the students, favourable and appropriate perceptions will
be formed. One can see this at work in the now widely-used system
of allowing each student to provide total nursing care for the
patients in her care for a period of time. The students form a more
personally satisfying picture of nursing as a process. Previously
acquired knowledge influences our perception of events in that it
provides frames of references against which current information is
judged. We perceive things as we know them to be, not necessarily
as they are. This can be demonstrated visually. When we look at
a house in the distance and we see a small house – say half an inch
high – surrounded by trees two inches high, we are not fooled into
perceiving them as small. The rest of the distant landscape
provides a frame of reference that enables us to make fairly accurate judgments of their size. We have changed our frames of
reference from the immediate vicinity to the distant one. Although
in a given society there will be similar frames of reference about
general things, acquired from initiation into a common culture,
there are always differences between people because experiences are
personal and largely unique. The present writer has no experience
in microbiology and could not tell the difference between bacilli
and cocci if he saw them. An expert in the field could be expected
not only to classify them correctly but would also know what to
do about them.

Sometimes different people have conflicting frames of reference
that can lead to problems of understanding. A ward sister may
perceive the student who spends a lot of time chatting to a
particular patient as wasting her time when there is work to do,
whilst the student may see herself as legitimately practising her
'social interaction skills', and attending to the psychological needs
of the patient.

Frames of reference are the means by which we classify and
categorise events in our perceptual field and form the basis of our
judgments and consequent action. The purpose of learning,
according to cognition theories, is to construct a number of organised detailed frames of reference held in a sufficiently flexible way
to enable us to change from one to another when considering an
event or problem so that the best judgment is made and a rational
course of action is taken. In order to understand how this happens
we need to understand two ideas that are central to cognition
theory. The first is 'concepts' and the other 'cognitive structures'.

A concept is the idea of something. It is an abstraction of the common properties or attributes of similar things. For example: bed, patient, ward, nurse, are all concepts in that they refer to classes of things, not single instances. It is not the word that is meant here but the idea denoted by it. The term 'patient' refers to a class of things containing numerous instances or examples all of whom have some things in common, and some things that are different. The things they have in common, or critical attributes, are the things that help us to define a concept, which in turn helps us to identify further examples of that class of things. One presumes the concept 'patient' may be defined as: 'a sick person in receipt of medical or nursing treatment'. Concepts are formed from numerous percepts of similar things, and are the way by which we deal with the millions of percepts we form daily. Without some form of simplication of this kind we would never be able to cope with out lives, nor think, nor communicate with others.

Not all concepts refer to concrete things: some like love, pride, time and weight are abstract. Some are simple, like 'patient', with only a few critical attributes, whilst others such as 'emotion', 'perception' and 'learning are complex.

The same process by which we simplify and organise sensations into percepts, and percepts into concepts, also enables us to organise concepts into hierarchies or cognitive structures. For example: 'dog' belongs to a family called canis, the family canis belongs to a class of mammals, which in turn are vertebrates, which are animals. Each group becomes more inclusive the further we move up the hierarchy. People differ in the content of their hierarchies. In the above examples, some may have dog – mammal – animal as the only categories, whilst others may have extensive structures linked and merged laterally. Hierarchies in anatomy may be cross-linked with those in the class of physiology. The differences in organisation are said to be due to innate ability, and the kind of experience received.

The value of concepts and cognitive structures is that they enable us to classify events and to make judgments and (unlike repertoires of behaviours and lists of facts) enable us to solve new problems. If the process of nursing is seen as a problem-solving activity in which the nurse acts on her own intitiative generating her own solutions, rather than one in which she repeats ready-made solutions; and if the reasoning of the cognition theorists is accepted as valid; then the teaching of nursing should be organised in such a way that the student not only acquires the necessary knowledge and skills, but does so in such a way that they develop in her flexible cognitive structures.

Associative and cognitive theories present two major examples of different approaches to the study of learning, and although they differ in very many respects it is possible to synthesise them in a way that offers guidance for teachers. Gagné's hierarchy of learning types brings together simple and complex forms of learning in a logical way, providing a model for planning and sequencing learning.

Conditions of learning

As the process of learning is hidden, it is not accessible to direct influence; however, it is possible for the teacher to do more than tell the student what she needs to learn. Within the constraints and limitations of the ward, the teacher can arrange and structure teaching to facilitate learning. This facilitation involves meeting conditions necessary for learning to take place.

Some of these conditions are internal to the learner, e.g. motivational states, attitudes, intelligence; others are under the direct control of the teacher and consist of ways of structuring teaching. Four of these, considered by Gagné as basic to all learning, are:

1. Contiguity
2. Practice
3. Feedback
4. Readiness.

Contiguity

Contiguity refers to the simultaneous occurrence of stimuli and responses in learning. In the classical conditioning experiment, the two stimuli were presented simultaneously. Operant conditioning involves contiguity, in that the reinforcing event follows closely the production of a response. Contiguity is necessary in all forms of learning.

Practice

Practice is the repetition of responses and is necessary for learning to become permanent. It is more important in simpler forms of learning such as skill learning when it usually means repetition. In complex learning such as problem-solving, it can mean having the opportunity to perform further activities within a particular class of problems.

Feedback

The third necessary condition is the provision of various forms of feedback to the student. During the process of learning the student is working to achieve something; knowledge of how close her performance is approximating to the desired goal not only has a motivating effect, but if given in sufficient detail provides information which enables her to adjust her learning nearer to the goal. In the early stages of learning a task, feedback in the form of words such as 'good' and 'well done' should be provided more frequently and immediately. Errors too should be pointed out immediately, so that they can be corrected before they have become established.

Later, as the student becomes more proficient, she will provide her own feedback and the teacher may delay or withhold comments. Setting intermediate goals and providing an assessment of them is another way that feedback can help the student adjust her learning. The ideal end state is reached when the student can accurately assess her own performance, but this will only occur after periods of meeting externally set requirements.

Readiness to learn

The final set of conditions we shall consider can be represented by the term 'readiness to learn'. By this is meant that the student must have the prerequisite knowledge and skills to begin learning the task. All too often students have difficulty or fail in their learning because they have an imperfect grasp of some concept, or because they have not learned some particular skill. Gagńe has provided a formula by which we may detect what is missing from a student's repertoire. It also provides a structure that links together different types of learning in a logical way and can provide a structure for planning and sequencing learning. Types of learning are distinguished, and are arranged in an hierarchical way so that earlier types are necessary conditions for later types of learning. The final type is the solving of problems. Categories are as follows:

1. *Sign learning*

2. *Stimulus–response learning*
3. *Chaining*.

These three types were described under associative learning. In sign learning, the student makes diffuse responses to signals in the environment. In type two, specific behaviours are linked with specific events as in classical and operant conditioning. In type three, the responses are linked in sequences or chains as in performing a motor skill.

4. Verbal learning. The learner acts appropriately on receiving verbal instructions or requests. This requires that the student understands the terms used, especially technical terms. Without this understanding further learning is restricted.

5. Discrimation learning. The student learns to recognise and distinguish between different kinds of events and responds to them appropriately.

Examples:

> The student identifies different signs and symptoms, distinguishes abnormal breathing from normal, distinguishes between the onset of pressure sores and normal skin, and discriminates between examples of infected, socially clean and sterile dressings.

Discrimination learning is facilitated by the use of the correct technical terms (verbal learning).

6. Concept learning. Whereas in discrimination learning the student learns to distinguish between events and objects on the basis of their differences, in concept learning she concentrates on the similarities of phenomena belonging to a class and makes a common response to them.

Examples:

> Responds appropriately to different signs of internal and external haemorrhage.
> Employs aseptic techniques in different situations. Defines asepsis.

7. Rule learning. Rules are combinations or chains of concepts which guide and regulate practice.

Examples:

> Haemorrhage reduces cardiac output.
> After a period of peripheral circulatory failure there is a danger of renal failure.
> Aseptic techniques require sterile equipment.

8. Problem Solving. The student recalls the relevant concepts, rules and skills and combines them to form a solution to a problem.

Examples:

> How can we change this patient's dressing without risking infection?
> This patient has suffered a period of acute hypoxia.
> What are the dangers, what signs should we look for? What action can we take?

Readiness to learn can be seen as the possession of learning at lower levels of the hierarchy, necessary to begin learning the present task.

We can now look at some applications of these principles to teaching.

Learning psychomotor skills

A large percentage of nursing consists of actions which, when analysed, can be seen as skills. It is not surprising, therefore, that much of the clinical teacher's time is spent in teaching combinations of a variety of skills. We shall now review skill learning.

A skill has three characteristics:

1. It is a chain of muscular movements called motor responses.
2. It involves the co-ordination of hand and eye movements.
3. It requires the organisation of chains into a complex response pattern.

A chain is a sequence of stimulus and response units. After the initial stimulus, which is usually an intention to commence the action, the completion of a response acts as the stimulus for subsequent responses, so that the chain becomes a smooth action. An example of a chain can be seen when starting a car which can be plotted as follows:

S (intent to start engine)	R (looking forward and to rear)
S (sight of clear road)	R (testing gear for neutral)
S (gear in neutral)	R (turning key)
S (sound of engine firing)	R (release of key)
S (key released)	R (depress accelerator)

Not only does this action involve hand–eye co-ordination but it also involves information received by the other senses. For this reason, skills are sometimes called perceptual-motor skills. Most nursing skills consist of a number of chains or subtasks combined to make up a complex response pattern. It seems that the subtasks are arranged hierarchically and that learning follows the sequence from small or simple elements to chains and sequences.

Skill learning falls into three phases: cognitive, fixation and autonomous.

During the cognitive phase, students attempt to intellectualise the skill and form a verbal plan which guides execution. During the fixation phase, the correct sequences are practised until the chances of making errors are reduced and the behaviour becomes fixed. This may take days, months or years in some cases.

The autonomous phase is characterised by the disappearance of the verbal plan and an increase in speed and accuracy. The skill becomes increasingly resistant to stress influences and can be continued despite outside interference. No conscious effort is required, and it is sometimes possible to carry on a non-relevant activity, e.g. holding a conversation, whilst performing the activity. Once this phase has been reached, forgetting is unlikely.

We can turn now to the application of the basic learning conditions.

Contiguity

In skill learning this means the proper sequencing and timing of the elements of a chain. There are two possible variations in sequencing. The skill can be learned as a whole and in the same sequence as normally performed in practice. This is best for complex and highly organised skills where component parts interact. The whole method is a form of simplification.

In less organised skills where there is little interaction, subtasks may be learned and practised separately before combining them.

Practice

Practice serves to strengthen the S–R elements of the chain, to aid the learning of sequences, to prevent forgetting and to strengthen the fixation and autonomous phases. Periods of practice should be spaced with short rest periods in between, but much will depend on the time available and the opportunities provided on the ward.

Feedback

Feedback is especially important in skill learning. Two forms have been delineated: extrinsic and intrinsic.

Extrinsic feedback is provided by the teacher in the form of information about the success or failure of the practice to match up to the standard performance. It must be provided immediately to have any effect on learning: the longer the delay, the slower the rate of learning. Intrinsic feedback is obtained through the student's own actions and is of two kinds – internal and external.

Internal or kinaesthetic feedback is the feeling obtained from the muscles when performing a skill. It is that 'right feel' about an action that tells one all is well. It may take some time before a beginner experiences it, but performance will not become efficient until she does.

External feedback is information obtained through the senses, usually visually, by which the student can judge the level of performance and make corrections where necessary.

An extension of intrinsic feedback is the feeling of satisfaction obtained after completing a skill successfully.

Extrinsic feedback from the teacher is necessary during skill learning and early practice, until intrinsic feedback takes over.

The final set of conditions for successful skill learning are derived from the learning hierarchy. It is necessary for the teacher to ensure that the student can perform any prerequisite skills, can make any discriminations and possesses the concepts and rules required during performance. For example, in learning to prepare and give an injection, has the student sufficient knowledge of aseptic technique? Can she measure in the appropriate units?

We can now draw up a simple plan for teaching a skill:

1. Analyse the skill, breaking it down into S–R units, chains, subtasks, prerequisite knowledge and skills.
2. Assess complexity of skill and decide whether to use part or whole method.
3. Determine whether the student has the prerequisite knowledge and skills. This is usually done by questioning to assist recall. Arrange training for anything not known.
4. Demonstrate and describe the skill, emphasising important parts.
5. Help student devise a verbal plan.
6. Provide for contiguity and reinforced practice.
7. Provide extrinsic feedback.
8. Help student to notice intrinsic feedback.
9. Provide remedial practice for parts with which the student is having difficulty.

Learning knowledge

Knowledge is understood to consist of facts and concepts combined into hierarchies of rules, the purpose of which is to inform and guide practice so that not only will nursing be more efficient but also professional problems not previously encountered by the nurse can be solved. This is a higher use of knowledge and is called generalisation.

To achieve this the nurse needs more than facts and skills; she needs the capabilities represented by the higher levels of the learning hierarchy. We shall now review these higher levels.

Discrimination learning

Discrimination learning is especially important for nursing practice as nurses are constantly faced with distinguishing between one set of conditions and another in the form of signs and symptoms, in the form of differences in kinds of equipment and their use, and in the form of differences in patients' problems and needs.

Two difficulties often encountered in this type of learning are: that complex phenomena are more difficult to distinguish than simple ones, and when similar phenomena, that is those with many characteristics in common, are being examined there is a greater chance of confusion. To help the learner, complex examples should be reduced to the essential characteristics and differences emphasised.

The basic conditions apply in that discrimination learning requires that the early levels of the hierarchy have been satisfactorily acquired in relation to the current events being discriminated.

Contiguity refers to ensuring that the student has the opportunity to make suitable responses. Practice is interpreted as repetition, and feedback consists mainly of approving reactions from the teacher.

Concept and rule learning

Both discrimination learning and concept learning are related to and dependent on the process of perception as described earlier, but both concept and rule learning have a close affinity with language. Concepts and rules are most often taught by definition and description, and whilst this can be successful, given a good communication technique, it has the disadvantage of failing to produce generalisation. But in the clinical area it is possible to teach concepts by observation and experiences supported by language. The following plan is one way that this can be achieved:

1. The student is informed of what she will be expected to do after she has learned the concept. This will be the identification of new examples of the concept.
2. The teacher ensures by questioning or other means that the student can make necessary discriminations and has knowledge of the appropriate terminology.
3. The teacher presents positive and negative examples of concept. A positive example is one that has the necessary attributes whilst a negative one has none. The latter are useful in that they shorten the time taken to learn the concept. Several of both kinds are needed, depending on the student, and are presented either simultaneously or in alternate sequence over a period of time.
   During this learning period the teacher should encourage the student to talk about the examples, and in the early stages ways should be found to make the essential characteristics stand out.
4. Testing is carried out by presenting the student with a new example of the concept and asking her to identify it. If she does this correctly she has learned the concept.

The teaching of rules, which are combinations of concepts, consists mainly of assisting the student to recall those involved, ensuring that they are fully understood and combined in the right order, and in providing the opportunities in clinical practice to apply them. It follows then that when the student can correctly apply the rule in a variety of situations, she can be said to have learned the rule.

In considering problem-solving, the final level of the hierarchy, it is necessary to distinguish between the learning of solutions and learning how to solve problems. When teaching theatre nursing, in the accident and emergency department and in other situations where teaching is dictated by the medical condition of the patient, the student is learning established solutions to problems. Teaching is almost always by the expository method of demonstration and description, and the kind of learning involved is at a lower level of the hierarchy. Learning how to solve problems is a more complex activity in that it involves thinking at a higher level. To solve a problem the student must recall the relevant concepts and rules and combine them in a way that satisfies the principles of good practice. This can be taught, in that the teacher can create the optimum conditions for this kind of learning. The most satisfactory way of teaching problem-solving is by the method of guided discovery, in which the teacher presents the problem usually in the form of a question. The student formulates her solution which is checked by the teacher and, where circumstances allow, carries out the solution. In the final discussion stage, the student evaluates her work.

The degree of complexity of the problem chosen will depend on the level of the student.

The steps for creating this kind of learning are as follows:

1. Present the problem, usually in the form of a question, and indicate the form the solution will take but not the solution itself.
2. Assist the recall of the relevant concepts, rules and skills involved in the solution.
3. Guide the students, according to their experience, through the process of formulating and testing hypotheses by indicating which areas to focus on.
4. Check the solution.
5. Supervise the application where necessary.
6. Encourage final self-evaluation.

Unusual questions, ideas and solutions from the student should be treated with respect. In the early stages a higher proportion of errors will occur, but these should be shown to have value in the process of reaching a solution. Opportunities should be created where time allows, for self-initiated learning.

This form of teaching takes more time than other methods but the emphasis is on learning the processes of thinking and organisation involved in reaching solutions. By ensuring the student has the prerequisite knowledge and skills, the time involved can be reduced considerably.

Conclusion

In this chapter we have reviewed some types of learning and the conditions necessary to promote them. How far the teacher will be able to meet these conditions will depend on the constraints imposed by the ward, how periods of clinical experience are viewed by tutorial and clinical staff and what kind of learning the teacher wishes to promote in the student; and this depends, very much, on how the teacher views the process of nursing.

REFERENCES

Gagne, R. M. (1970) *The Conditions of Learning*. New York: Holt Rinehart & Winston.

Walker, S. (1975) *Learning and Reinforcement*. London: Methuen.

FURTHER READING

Abercrombie, M. L. J. (1967) *The Anatomy of Judgement*. London: Hutchinson.

Borger, R. & Seaborne, A. E. M. (1966) *The Psychology of Learning*. Harmondsworth: Penguin.

De Cecco, J. & Crawford, W. (1974) *The Psychology of Learning and Instruction*. Hemel Hempstead Prentice-Hall.

Gregory, R. (1966) *Eye and Brain: The Psychology of Seeing*. London: Weidenfeld & Nicholson.

Hilgard, E. R. & Bower, G. H. (1975) *Theories of Learning*. Hemel Hempstead: Prentice-Hall.

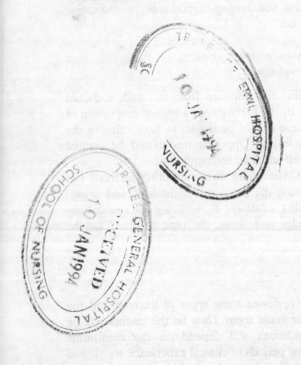

6

Teaching resources

'You cannot teach a man anything, you can only help him to find it within himself'.   Galileo.

Education today, both in the general educational field and in nurse education, involves the use of a vast array of differing materials and equipment (software and hardware); and the use of an expanse of knowledge, in the form of libraries, journals, and research documents. In this chapter on teaching resources, I shall endeavour to aid the reader in the selection and use of materials, production of handouts, worksheets and visual aids, as well as understanding a wider look at resources.

Teaching is the ability to communicate effectively to the student or pupil, enabling learning to take place. Teaching or learning resources are tools that enable the communication to be more effective. Only by increasing the motivation of the student, increasing attention, and aiding attainment of knowledge, skills and desirable attitudes, will learning take place, causing a permanent change in behaviour. Teaching aids must not be introduced solely in order to save time, but must make possible an increase in understanding for the learner. Assessment of any visual aid must be based on its ability to convey information, and therefore differing types of media are required for differing teaching methods.

Students today are used to visual effects of a high quality, such as in documentary programmes on television, and expect competence on behalf of the tutor and clinical teacher in their use.

In 1971, the General Nursing Council convened a committee to look into the the use of visual aids in training schools. The report highlighted the under-utilisation of expensive equipment. Similar findings were found by Marson of Sheffield Polytechnic with the under-use of programmed material and visual aids. (Marson 1971, Townsend 1975).

115

The role of the teacher is changing, with less emphasis on the teacher providing all the material for the student, but increased emphasis on providing a stimulating environment for active learning to take place. During primary education, the child learns by two methods:

1. Doing (play) – using resources provided.
2. Being told – verbal communication by the parent and teacher.

During secondary education, the use of the spoken word increases. It is economical in time and resources, but sadly is only effective if the teacher is one of the rare breed who is highly skilled in lecturing methods. *Telling is not teaching*. Owing to shortage of teachers in nurse education, and the number of learners, we are gradually returning to learning by discovery, with the teacher acting as guide, counsellor and facilitator – in other words, the learner is *doing*. Resources are the hub of this method of education, in which books, programmed texts, tape-slides, ERIC micro-fiche, charts, dissection of organs, research documents and patients' care plans are all used in the learning process. Discussion and evaluation take place with the tutor, enabling individual assistance to the learners, according to their special needs.

The learning resources centre serves teachers and learners alike. In many teaching establishments, a media resources officer is available to give advice on equipment, materials, maintenance of equipment and production of visual and audio aids. The teacher, librarian and media officer need to understand each other's special skills in order to work together as a team:

1. The teacher analyses the learning needs;
2. The media officer translates them into the design;
3. The librarian obtains the information and resources.

The final decision must be the teacher's. Not all schools of nursing are so well equipped or staffed as to afford a media officer, and responsibility for the care and maintenance of equipment is delegated to teaching staff. Related to nursing, the term 'teaching resources' includes the entire hospital personnel, the equipment of the hospital, the primary care team in the community, the patient and his family.

Team-teaching is another term which needs introduction. It can include the immediate team of tutors and clinical teachers within the school of nursing, but in the wider sense it includes the medical staff and all trained staff of wards and departments, each with their special skills, personalities and valuable experience. Allocation of time and facilities with ample free time for discussion is essential for effective team teaching. Success will depend upon each individual contribution and the effort put into the teaching programme, coupled with the ability to work in harmony. The sum total should be far greater than each individual component. Good communication within the team is essential for harmonious working relationships, with weekly meetings headed by the team leader to discuss the nurses' evaluation of their modular experiences. The knowledge, skills and desirable attitudes to be encouraged, translated into team objectives, form the core of the team approach. This translation is tedious but essential work, as the nurse and the team must both know in which direction they are to proceed. A final evaluation based on the objectives follows at the completion of each module. Each module should include objectives indicating aspects of care related to the changing needs of society:

1. Pattern of disease health problems,
2. Expectation of health,
3. Patient and family needs.

In this way the curriculum objectives become a teaching resource, upon which the method of teaching and selection of teaching aids are based.

The learner as a resource person

Nursing care based upon the nursing process is being widely implemented in the United Kingdom, and one of the main skills that nurses need to develop is the ability to be able to communicate effectively with the patient and his family, in order to be able to define the patient's problems. Communication within the caring team, and the formation of nursing care plans, ensures continuity of patient care. In the past, it has been assumed that nurses have already developed these skills when leaving school, or that they are acquired whilst providing patient care. LeLean (1973) and Ashworth (1980) both identify the need to include interpersonal skills in the nursing curriculum. Nurses tend to control most patient/nurse conversations, and therefore may ignore what the patient needs to discuss. Most questions that nurses ask patients are closed questions, and therefore do not encourage the patient to express his feelings of social, emotional, or physical need.

The learner may be regarded as a resource person by encouraging intercommunication between learners in role playing, and experiential learning, which are then followed by discussion and analysis of the effectiveness of the situation enacted, and the feelings which were generated towards each other. Abbott Laboratories Ltd (see p. 148) have produced a learning package of video-tapes concerned with the elderly and the patient with cancer. The presentation contains guidance for the tutor to enable maximum learning and skill development. Tutors may like to venture further and produce their own 'situational' tapes covering aspects of ward management and patient care. Many articles have been written on communication skills, which may assist with ideas. The Nursing Bibliography produced by the Royal College of Nursing is essential for every nursing library, both for tutors and learners, when exploring areas for study. Discussion also assists learners to identify their own feelings and attitudes, so deepening understanding of themselves, their patients and colleagues. Clamp (1980) sets out eight objectives which may be achieved by learning through incidents, and these briefly are to be able to:

1. analyse work
2. identify and describe feelings and behaviour
3. demonstrate empathy
4. identify problems and make decisions
5. demonstrate intellectual skills, verbal skills, the ability to think
6. discuss how understanding of patients, relatives and colleagues as individuals can be achieved
7. explain the concept of a harmonious team
8. assist peers and colleagues more positively.

When one works with learners in the ward, discussion of all aspects of communication, including non-verbal communication, is essential. What did the learner do well? What does she need to improve? When one provides any care, whether it is managing a group of patients, or bathing one patient, the following skills are demonstrated – social skills, management skills, communication skills, and practical skills. When one gives the learner feedback on her ability these skills provide a framework for assessment. Patients experience high anxiety levels at time of admission to hospital. Why did the learner not identify the signs of anxiety expressed through non-verbal behaviour? How could the anxiety have been avoided? What lessons are to be learned and applied to future care? These are skills which can be simulated in the classroom, but teacher and learner need to work through situations together in the real world, so that learner can receive the support she needs. This could later provide the basis for a role play or discussion session in the classroom.

In the clinical area, learners develop their practical and social skills, but at the same time develop a full sense of responsibility, especially if given the guidance and support they need to become safe and competent practitioners. Teaching, too, becomes teaching for reality, so narrowing the gap between theory and practice (Bendall, 1976).

Nursing research as a teaching resource

If nursing is to become a profession, it needs to develop its own body of knowledge. Nurses providing care in the community or hospital, and teachers planning the curriculum, must base practice upon theory (i.e. a body of knowledge) that has been researched. This body of nursing knowledge is growing rapidly, and trained nurses should be encouraging learners to question what they do, and why. Is the care effective? Could the care be improved? Has any study been made of a similar problem? The librarian may be able to carry out a relevant literature search. Nursing care can run the risk of becoming ritualised. We do things like this because we have always done it that way. This care is not necessarily unsafe or ineffective, but we should always ask whether there is a more effective method, and in some cases, whether we need to do it at all.

For research to become a learning resource, lists of suggested reading in preparation for modules of experience should contain reference to relevant nursing research, in order to prepare for discussion in class. This gives learners guidance in their self-directed learning, and encourages a problem-solving approach to care. A problem-solving approach is a necessary feature of the nursing process, in which it is applied to seek to alleviate the patient's problems; it is also crucial to the research process.

In the final year of training, investigative projects can be given to learners as intermodular work, and the presentation of such projects can form part of their modular assessment. Some of the topics which might be suggested to learners are:

- Handwashing techniques – application and efficacy
- Accuracy of fluid charts – are they always necessary?
- Standards for recording observations of vital signs

- Advice to patients before discharge
- Catheter care and the incidence of urinary infection
- Oral hygiene – methods and effectiveness of care
- Support for junior nurses – what are their needs?
- How could senior students better assist them?

The ward sister naturally needs to be consulted, and this can be discussed at a preliminary interview between the learner and the sister. The tutor and clinical teacher can give guidance and support to ensure that too large a topic is not undertaken: 'advice to patients before discharge' needs to be narrowed to an area of care which is part of the modular experience. A literature search has to be made by the learner, who then makes an assessment of the particular problem. The project should include a review of the literature, a summary of the findings relating to the aspect of care investigated, and suggestions for improving care based on the investigation. These projects encourage a questioning attitude, and the application of nursing research findings to patient care by the ward team. When presenting the project, learners can be encouraged to use audio-visual aids, and to view the exercise as valuable experience in the development of their own teaching skills. Project topics should be organised by the tutor prior to presentation so that a logical sequence can be developed, aiding discussion by the total group. Teacher and learner learn together. Ward staff are invited and encouraged to participate in the learner's project and to attend the presentation. When compiling the timetable, a time should be selected to enable the maximum number of trained staff to attend.

Knowledge is never static, but successive generations of nurses fail to implement the findings of research. Why is this so if the curriculum is to be based on research? Very little research has been carried out on teaching methods and the effectiveness of learning in nurse education. Lectures feed learners with information, giving them a feeling of security because they have notes which they may then be able to regurgitate when answering a theoretical question. But how much of this knowledge is applied in the ward? Eve Bendall (1976) in 'Teaching for reality' states that '. . . the major part of written answers to nursing questions bear little or no relationship to the nursing performance of the writer in 80% of trainees', and she goes on to say '. . . we are producing trained nursing staff who are (through no fault of their own) woefully lacking in many of the skills they need.' It seems from this work that theory and practice must be directly linked, and the main area in which to teach these linkages is the clinical area.

Learners when questioned about why an aspect of nursing care is necessary often demonstrate poor understanding of the principles upon which such care is based, in relation to their patient's need. If learners were encouraged to be more active in the learning process, rather than sitting in a classroom, and this active learning was based on patient care in the clinical area, would the learning be more realistic? Self-directed learning takes a great deal of planning by the teaching team, and teachers are reluctant to let go of the responsibility of being the main teaching resource. Learners, too, can become very anxious if they are not fully supported during their learning experience.

The development of a problem-solving, self-directed course of study

'Patient problems' provide a basis for studying nursing, and so these problems form the presenting, or trigger, problems which are given to the learners. The material is discussed and analysed in order to identify what it is necessary to know in order to solve the problem, and hence manage patient care. The curriculum content is based upon problems in differing areas of patient care, and nurses with specialist skills and experience are necessary to construct the curriculum and programme evaluation.

A presenting 'problem' to the learner might be, for example:

1. 'Difficulty in breathing': The tutor and learners decide what they need to know in order to understand the problem and provide nursing care. How do we all breathe normally? How is breathing controlled? How can nursing skills assist breathing? How does medical treatment reduce the problem?
2. 'Difficulty in expectoration' may be another problem. What is sputum? How is it produced and why? What is infection and its effect on the respiratory tract? How can nursing care and physiotherapy aid expectoration? What medical care and treatment will reduce the patient problem?
3. 'Confusion' may be another associated problem. Why does confusion occur? How does the nurse manage the confused patient? What are the advantages and dangers of oxygen administration? Does the patient smoke? How do you ensure patient safety?
4. 'Difficulty with eating and drinking': What is the importance

of ensuring fluid and energy intake, especially in a pyrexial patient? What are the complications of dehydration, and those of poor oral hygiene?

Many other problems may be presented, for example problems related to preparing the patient for safe discharge to the community. The examples stated here are basic to all patients with a respiratory problem, or problem of the cardiovascular system. However, the cause of the problem in a particular patient will be different, and so actual care may also differ. If the learner can be guided through the programme, and can begin to delineate for herself what she needs to know, then the knowledge and skills developed should become more relevant and an inquiring attitude should be strengthened in the learner.

The timetable for this form of learning needs to be much less formal. Planned tutorials or lectures can be programmed for material which might provide a basis for development. The use of reading lists, tapes, slides, video-recordings etc. needs to be carefully planned, because they form a major resource. The tutor is the facilitator of learning, and the learner is active. The workshops mentioned later in the chapter may provide a hub for the self-directed learning by basing them on the problem(s). Suggested steps in the planning are as follows, and it will be immediately apparent that they take time:

1. Prepare outline (broad) aims and objectives for period of study.
2. Identify 'problems' for study according to learners' current ward allocation.
3. Decide on the order of the presentation of material to the learner and produce flow diagrams.
4. Prepare objectives for nursing care based on patient problems.
5. Circulate objectives and outline course material to all concerned (ward staff particularly) for discussion.
6. Make modifications and prepare a breakdown of study programme into learning units, demonstrating how the patient 'problems' fit into the units.
7. Prepare trigger material to be presented to the learner:
   (i) Worksheet, reading list, audiovisual aids etc.
   (ii) Prepare flow guide for tutors who will support learners through the process of problem-solving in order to attain the expected outcomes.
8. Ensure that all objectives can be met by the programme provided.

9. Prepare assessment instrument based on objectives, and circulate for comments. This might include continuous assessment of the learner in the clinical area, with the expected level of competence defined in the objectives, appropriate to the learners' stage of training.
10. Make alterations following discussion.
11. Design an evaluation sheet for tutors and learners.
12. Revise unit material on the basis of the evaluation.

Learners need to see the total experience (theory and practice) as a learning module, and many of the topics explored are discovered, discussed, and learned as a result of caring for the patient. What? Why? How? When? need to be asked constantly by the learner.

The dual role of the learner as a student and employee causes conflict in the clinical area between the need to learn and the multiple pressures exerted upon all ward staff committed to patient care. Bendall (1976) states '. . . the most fundamental mistake was to separate those who teach and those who practise.' As a result of this separation, and the increased pressures upon the nurse teacher and the ward sister, theory and reality have sometimes drifted apart. I have suggested a way of learning which uses the skills of both the teacher and the trained nurse in the clinical environment, working together to improve patient care. Nurses should become more knowledgeable, and able to apply such knowledge to patient care, and encourage the development of professional competence in the delivery of individualised care to patients.

Why do we need teaching aids?

The term 'aid' is very often coupled with 'audio-visual' and 'learning'. Aid means help, but often aids are learning materials in their own right, e.g. programmed texts. The primary goal of audio-visual instruction is learning, and, through research, techniques have been developed to enrich learning.
There are three main levels of providing learning experiences.

1. The closer one can get to reality, the easier the learning by the student, provided that the necessary knowledge has been given previously to facilitate comprehension.
2. Learning through audio-visual materials, i.e. objects, specimens, modules, slides, filmstrips, radio and television. Although they do not provide the real experience, they aid and increase understanding and motivation.

3. Learning through the use of words, e.g. speech, writing, formulae, used singly or in combination for discussion, presentation of seminars, projects, essays etc.

The general value of teaching aids is:

1. To enrich learning and add dynamic interest.
2. To increase understanding of concepts.
3. To increase acquisition of knowlege and aid retention of factual information.
4. To provide a stimulus for discussion.
5. To encourage voluntary reading.
6. To motivate students by allowing them to share a common experience.
7. To foster desirable attitudes and change behaviour.
8. to allow experts into the classroom.
9. To expand the social and physical environment of the learner.

Teaching aids are therefore valuable for students of all ages and experience.

Availability and selection of aids

In these days of financial restraint, the availability of teaching aids and the more expensive equipment may be limited by the budget. However, much can be done by the teachers themselves at very little cost to the department. A little thought and ingenuity is all that is required. Very often, the simpler the aid the more effective it is, and less likely to go wrong.

The following points should be borne in mind:
1. Any visual aid should be carefully selected and planned to add clarity to the presentation.
2. The rationale for using the aid is:
   a. To simulate reality.
   b. To increase retention.
   c. To increase motivation.
   d. To stimulate discussion.
   e. To demonstrate relationships.
3. Would any other type of aid be more effective or appropriate?
4. Are visual movement or tactile stimuli necessary?
5. Is the visual display area adequate?
6. Is there an electricity supply?

7. Is it cheaper in the long term to buy rather than to hire?
8. Is the aid reliable and in working order?
9. Commercially produced films, tape-slide presentations and programmed texts must be viewed in advance. Catalogues describing films can be misleading about the information they contain. The content may be too trivial or too deep for the group, causing embarrassment to the teacher. Students are not reluctant to hide their frustration and impatience.
10. Each individual piece of equipment has a special contribution to make; for example, a tape recorder can be equally effective in stimulating discussion as a film, but films or video tapes are more effective for the demonstration of practical skills where movement is essential.
11. When selecting equipment to buy, one should make sure that servicing facilities are good and spare parts are quickly obtainable. How long would servicing take? Is there a replacement service for equipment, or can one hire similar equipment from within one's area? If equipment has to travel between hospitals and schools, it must be able to withstand stress and so a strong carrying case is preferable. This seems obvious, but is not always heeded when selecting items.
12. When any equipment is purchased, an account of the cost of software (paper, film, video-tape, slides) must also be included.
13. How many staff can use the equipment? Will special instructions be required for most of the staff, in order that the materials can be fully utilised, or will it be the 'toy' of one or two people; or will it lie dormant in a cupboard until someone revives interest in it?

In the *Journal of Advanced Nursing*, (1976) Marson and Townsend state that there is need for change in educational technology in this country. However, change of this nature is hindered by:

1. Lack of understanding about innovation.
2. Lack of the skills and knowledge needed to service equipment. This is particularly important when the installation of expensive equipment is contemplated.
3. Non-availability of the appropriate software.
4. Difficulties in organisational arrangements.
5. Lack of staff motivation.

Aids as teaching resources

1. Non-projected visual aids
    a. Pictorial –
        (i) Blackboard/whiteboard.
        (ii) Flip charts.
        (iii) Wall charts.
        (iv) Felt boards and Magnetic boards.
        (v) Noticeboards.
    b. 3-D Models.
    c. Simple visual aids for the teaching of principles and concepts.
2. Projected visual aids
    a. Overhead projector
        (i) Preparation of own material.
        (ii) Commercially produced material.
    b. Slides 2 cm × 2 cm and the slide projector.
    c. Epidiascope.
    d. Film loops.
    e. Films and film projector.
    f. Videotapes
3. Programmed Instruction
4. Audio aids
    a. Tape recorder.
    b. Radio.

Non-projected aids

This group of teaching aids is by far the most important, and should not be regarded as second rate. For clinical teaching, they can be fully mobile in many cases, and do not require an electricity supply. They are relatively cheap and sometimes can be produced by a hospital workshop – or an imaginative husband!

White board/chalk board. Very few classrooms are without this almost traditional teaching aid, and few teachers omit to use it. However, too often the student strains to see what is written because the teacher has not considered how she is using the board. Understanding the flexibility of this equipment leads to more efficient instruction.

All board work should be planned as far as possible when preparing the lesson, e.g.

Topic heading

Diagrams.   New Vocabulary.   Summary of Lesson.

One should decide whether any information would be better given on a hand-out, or on the overhead projector. The use of the board for superfluous material should be discouraged, since it should be used to make a learning sequence meaningful. Explanations of concepts and principles can be demonstrated by diagrams or verbally throughout the lesson. The summary may be retained, since headings of the lession plan usually make a good outline for students' notes. The rest of the board can be used for any material that may be erased.

Advantages of the chalkboard/whiteboard are:

1. It becomes an integral part of lesson planning, and the students can use the board to develop their own teaching expertise.
2. It is useful in recording progress in work programmes, e.g. trial and error ward management problems, one example of which might be organising patient allocation for total patient care and delegating responsibilities by senior student nurses. They would work in groups to present the final plan, showing the patients' needs and the nurses' needs. Evaluation of how the plan has met these needs takes place in open discussion in class.
3. Arrangement of ideas on the board provides a stimulus for new ideas and lateral thinking.
4. Project work can be developed in outline and the board allows for the planning and evaluation of group experiences.

When writing on the board, one should not carry on any verbal discussion, as the words are lost to the class. One should always face the students when addressing them.

Make sure that the written communication can be clearly seen.

1. Avoid glare on the board – shiny surfaces can be prevented by careful blackboard maintenance.
   Yellow chalk is sometimes better than white.
2. Do not stand in front of what you written.
3. Use the board calmly. Hurriedly written sentences are very often indecipherable. At a distance of 32 feet, letters must be $2\frac{1}{2}$ inches high to be clearly visible at the back of the class.
4. Make sure the board is clean on leaving the class.

Templates may be made by the teacher for outlines which are repeatedly used, e.g. the human body and its organs. These enable the production of more proficient diagrams by anyone who cannot draw. Cardboard or plywood can be used for this purpose.

Material may also be transferred to the board by making a

pattern of the diagram of the required size on paper. The outline is punched with small pinholes using a sewing tracing wheel. The pattern is then placed over the board, and the surface of the paper facing you is rubbed with chalk. On removing the paper from the board, an outline is produced as a series of small dots. During the lesson the diagram is drawn in when appropriate.

Another technique is to use the epidiascope to project the image onto the board and the picture can be outlined in coloured pencil. (Safe on rubberised boards only).

Whiteboards can be used similarly with watersoluble pens which enable the surface to be cleaned with a damp cloth. Care must be taken not to use spirit based pens as this makes cleaning impossible, except by using spirit. If this is not easily available, nobody will thank you for the error! The paper outline technique can still be used, but instead of chalk a light coloured pen can be used. It will just be visible to the teacher but not to the class. Projection onto the whiteboard is made directly, using the white surface as the screen.

Flip charts/Wall charts. The flip chart is a large pad of paper, which may be blank or filled with previously prepared diagrams, pictures, maps, cartoons and so on. There are commercially produced stands or easels to hold the papers, but a home-made version is cheap and easily stored. It can, furthermore, be used in the ward. The paper is clipped together by firm bulldog clips at the top edge of the required piece of hardboard, so allowing the charts to be turned over in an upwards direction. The stand must be free, that is, away from the wall and an intravenous stand would be ideal, particularly in the ward. For storage, the whole aid can be hung from the wall, or stored flat.

Each presentation may be a chart demonstrating relationships, a picture to stimulate discussion, or a series of sequences demonstrating a manipulative skill, procedure or physiological process. (Fig. 6.1).

To produce these pictures the paper must be fairly tough if they are to be kept. Sellotaping the edges will increase the life of the chart. Use cheaper paper if the communication is not to be retained. Drawing with thick felt pens is essential for the presentation to be clear. Use the epidiascope for outlining pre-prepared material as with the blackboard. Clear use of colour is also important. Above all else, the chart should:

1. Be simple – one should draw only that which is relevant.
2. Have a message.

3. Be attractive and not cluttered.
4. Use coloured pens or differing coloured backgrounds to increase attention.
5. Have letters large enough to be seen easily from a distance.

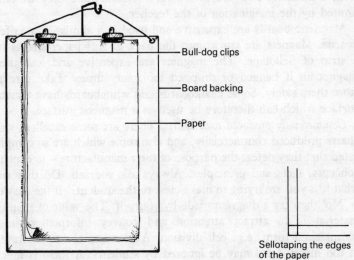

Bull-dog clips

Board backing

Paper

Sellotaping the edges of the paper

Fig. 6.1 A flip-chart.

Chart display. Classrooms, clinical rooms and seminar rooms are not always liberally equipped with hooks or pegs on which to hang charts. If you are fortunate, large soft boards are provided for the use of drawing-pins. Other methods are:

1. A long piece of cord/string by which charts can be suspended by a bulldog clip, paper clips or clothes pegs.
2. Plasticine, which will hold charts temporarily on a blackboard. The use of Plastitak or Blu-tack, which is similar, does not harm the wall.
3. Magnets which will hold charts with metal fittings to any metal strips or objects fixed to the wall.

Felt board/Magnet board display. Both these boards allow for movement of the display; they are therefore very good for the rearrangement of sequences, e.g. planning patient care, ward management, functions of the body, heart valves or types of joints. A homemade felt board is easily made from an old blanket. If the surface is brushed, making it fluffy, shapes cut from felt, flannel or material backed with flocked paper will easily adhere to the blanket. One can use paper shapes that are fairly stiff and stick a piece of Velcro on the back surface as this also sticks easily. Keep the pieces from each presentation in separate boxes, making re-use easy. They take time to make, but can be used many times. It is not time wasted. Make sure the presentation can be seen and read from a distance. Felt boards are very versatile, and they are only limited by the imagination of the teacher.

Magnetic boards are expensive and used in a similar way as felt boards. Magnets are stuck onto the back of stiff paper shapes by a strip of Sellotape. The magnets are expensive and lose their magnetism if banged or dropped too many times. Take care to store them safely. Some chalkboards and whiteboards have a metal surface which can therefore be used as a magnetic surface.

Commercially produced wall charts. There are some excellent wall charts produced commercially, and also some which are so complicated that they defeat the purpose of their manufacture – to explain concepts, facts and principles. Always ask yourself 'Do they say what it is you are trying to make clear to the student?' If the answer is 'No' then try a diagram made by yourself. The value of graphic material is to attract attention and convey information in a summarised form, e.g. cell division. Anatomical charts portrayed in too much detail may be ignored by students. A torso is much more effective in demonstrating relationships, because the learner is 'doing' by handling the organs, taking apart and putting them together again.

How to evaluate a wall chart:

1. Is the subject appropriately presented in this form?
2. Is the subject appropriate for the group?
3. Is it suitable for the level of the work?
4. For which purpose is it designed?
   a. To demonstrate skills?
   b. To show visual relationships?
   c. To organise knowledge?
   d. To stimulate and motivate learning?
   e. To modify and mould attitudes?
5. The design –
   a Is the message clear?
   b. Is the information easily obtained from the chart?
   c. Is the use of colour effective?
   d. Is the layout simple?
   e. Does it add to the communication which you are making?

Flat pictures. The versatility of the flat picture is enormous, and a collection of pictures from magazines and newspapers can be used to stimulate discussion. They can be pictures of situations, of people, places, facial expressions, or scenes of differing behaviour. Pasted to cardboard they can be stored.

Pictures are useful for interviewing purposes as not only do they assist discussion during a group interview, but they enable the interviewer to estimate the communication skills of the candidates. The level of understanding of people's needs and an estimation of the prospective nurse can be made from the discussion.

Pictures can be used to increase the powers of observation of nurses and the interpretation of non-verbal signals both to and from the patient. Scenes of ward situations enable the nurses to make a quick evaluation of a problem. How would they deal with the situation? What would their priorities be? The group can discuss the various interpretations. Would they have made a different assessment? Has the situation been dealt with effectively? Are there any legal or ethical problems arising from the depicted scene?

When choosing pictures for teaching, the teacher must have regard for the suitability of the picture and also consider whether the learner has the prerequisite knowledge to understand the picture. Has it interest value? Are the cues contained within the picture strong enough for their proper interpretation? What is the overall quality of the picture?

Posters. Posters must be kept simple, have a message, use colour subtly and be eyecatching. The design must captivate the audience. Used in workshops, they can add interest. In cartoon form they can very often clarify points, focusing upon topics that might otherwise be hurriedly overlooked as being too difficult to comprehend. A series of pictures depicting the formation of DNA using a train and trucks commences with something with which we are all familiar and can recall instantly.

Notice boards. Notice boards must be large enough to ensure that displayed items are not overlapping and obscuring one another. If the board is sectioned by coloured tape, and each section clearly headed (e.g. Introductory Course; Year 1; Year II; UKCC Royal College of Nursing notices), it makes selection of material to be read easier. Ideally, one person should be responsible for notice boards so that out-of-date notices are not cluttering the board and interest is maintained. Notice boards are meant to be noticed, and therefore must look attractive. Articles of up-to-date information will draw people to the board and encourage the use of a central information source. In this way they become a teaching resource.

Models

Models provide a three dimensional experience and very often a real understanding of the structure. They are made usually to be handled by the learner, but how often to you actually see nurses *using* the models? They are very often at the front of the class for the sole use of the teacher, whilst the class sits passively. Used in this way, a chart would probably be more effective because it may be larger and more easily seen at the back of the class. In workshops, learners should be encouraged to use the models effectively.

The size of commercially produced models for nurse education may be life size or greater. The principle of the model is to stimulate interest, but it does have its limitations. Provision of the real object where possible is usually eagerly explored. Dissection classes with small groups of students are excellent since even the squeamish can take part as onlookers, whilst a fellow student performs the dissection. An example of increasing learning is to dissect sheep's kidneys. Unless the outer capsule of fibrous tissue is actually felt by the learner, there is little appreciation of its strength and its protective function in maintaining the shape of the kidney. Similarly, an animal's eye can be easily dissected, but this would not increase understanding or explain the complex nervous system related to vision.

Models used to simulate resuscitation procedures are an invaluable aid, and enable the nurse to practice the skills of external cardiac massage and expired air ventilation; but however complete the simulation of the emergency situation, the emotional effects of the real situation cannot be taught. Ample discussion of these procedures and the ethical implications should be allowed in the timetable.

More complicated models for the simulation of cardiac arrhythmias are available for nurses specialising in intensive care work. The prerequisite knowledge of the cardiac cycle must be fully understood however, as must the 'normal' electrocardiogram.

Models to explain principles and concepts are usually welcomed by groups, particularly if biology and physics have not been studied in school. Examples that can be used are:

Two microscope slides can be placed together with water or oil between them to allow for easy movement across one another, but trying to pull them apart without sliding the surfaces together is very difficult. This demonstration helps in the understanding of a potential space (e.g. between the pleura).

Another example is the similarity of a piece of elastic to normal lung tissue and a piece of string to lung tissue in chronic chest conditions. The stretching of the elastic explains the elasticity of lung tissue and that energy is required to stretch the tissue. It is an active process. Release and recoil of the elastic is passive, no energy being required. The string demonstrates that energy is required to extend the string to its full length and that no elastic recoil is demonstrated on release of the string. Similarly in chronic chest disorders recoil is diminished, and only by using the accessory muscle of respiration is air expelled from the lungs.

The value of models is:
1. To simulate reality
2. To enable class participation, individually or in groups.
3. To complement worksheets and other teaching aids.
4. To give the learner visual, tactile and aural stimuli, which increase the learning experience.

In summary the model may be used as part of a learning sequence, so the teacher must ask the question 'has the learner the requisite knowledge and skills to enable further learning to take place?'

Exhibitions, visits etc. Visits are only as good as the preparation made before them. The exhibition or centre must be visited by teaching staff before the learners and an assessment made, which should include the following questions:

1. What are the aims and objectives of the visit?
2. Will the experience be of value to nurse education in its widest context?
3. What interest will be satisfied by the visit?
4. What preparation will be required?
5. Will the centre require knowledge of the needs of the nurses, so that they use the visit to their best advantage?
6. Do the learners need to spend more time in some areas than in others?
7. Is a worksheet necessary?
8. Can the group get to the centre easily?
9. What will the total cost be?
10. Will uniform or mufti be required?

Finally, allow time for discussion and evaluation of the visit.

Projected visual aids

Overhead projector. The overhead projector is probably the most used teaching aid after the blackboard/chalkboard. Indeed, it can sometimes be used as a board substitute but cannot entirely replace it. (The device projects onto a screen by passing light through an acetate sheet approximately 25 × 25 cm.)

Storage of transparencies allows them to be used at a later date, therefore time spent in careful production is time well used. Planning of the lesson sequence is important: what visual representations are required and what needs to be included on each transparency? Would a series of transparencies be better than overcrowding one frame?

The projector has many advantages: for instance, pre-production of the acetate sheet enables better layout, drawing and writing.

Transparencies can be studied for longer periods than drawings on the board, and no time is consumed by drawing during the lesson. However, there is a danger of giving too much information too quickly.

Additions can be made during the lesson by using permanent ink for the diagrams and using water-soluble pens for labels, which can be washed off later.

Intermittent use of the projector gives a change of teaching mode, thereby aiding and maintaining the interest of the class. The image is bright and the use of brightly coloured pens adds stimulus variation.

The teacher can face the class at all times, thereby alleviating the tendency to talk to the board. Highlighting important points is made *on* the projector, *not* on the screen. Use a sharp pointed instrument, such as a pen or pencil. If the finger is used, the image is partly obscured by the hand.

A further advantage of the projector is that it is cleaner to use than the chalkboard (Fig. 6.2).

Specialised uses:
1. Overlays can aid the build up of complex subjects.
2. Movement can be produced using silhouettes on the opaque screen.
3. Commercially produced transparencies are now more widely available.

Disadvantages of the overhead projector are few, and mainly relate to technical breakdown, such as a bulb blowing, or the fuse

The Overhead Projector

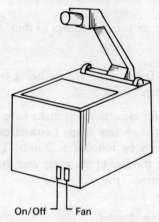

On/Off ⎯⎯ Fan

The Epidiascope

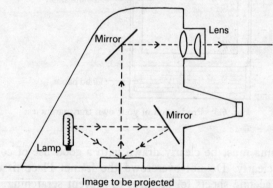

Fig. 6.2   The overhead projector and the epidiascope.

breaking. Some modern projectors have an inbuilt device for quickly switching to a new bulb. A broken one can be replaced at a more convenient time.

Making your own transparencies. There are three thicknesses of acetate:

0.004 of 2.5 cm	Flimsy
0.005 of "	Normal
0.007 of "	Thick

Use a thick piece of cardboard at least 30 cm × 30 cm square as a firm base to work on.
Use A4 or quarto paper with narrow lines (6 mm) as a guide for lettering.
Place acetate on the top.
Cover with a cardboard frame – the acetate being centralised.
Hold all in place with paper clips.

The lined paper allows for clear writing; make sure that all letters are the same height as the narrow lines. Letraset can be used, in which case the letters may be reduced to 3 mm. The size of the letters will depend upon the size of the room and the distance that the image is to be projected. (Fig. 6.3)

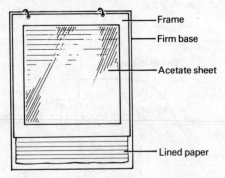

Fig. 6.3   Production of your own transparencies.

Diagrams must be clearly drawn with a good use of colour and labelled clearly. Do not overcrowd the frame. Place tissue paper between acetate sheets for storage, to prevent scratching.

Pens: Staedler – Lumicolour 315 washable ink pens (water soluble)
Staedler – lumicolour 317 pemanent ink pens (spirit soluble)
Staedler also make a fountain pen (cartridge) useful when using the projector for writing during the class.

Pentel also make a range of pens which are excellent, especially as the felt tips do not become fuzzy with use and maintain their firmness.

Washable and permanent ink pens can be used in conjunction with each other; for example, a diagram can be drawn in permanent ink and labelled in washable ink. This means that the labelling can be removed and the aid used as a recall test. A 'stock' of outlines, organs or microscopic structures of the body can be made in permanent ink. Movement of fluids, molecules, etc. can be illustrated as necessary using washable ink and then removed, allowing re-use of the basic diagram.

Evaluation tests and quick quizzes can be given using acetates on the projector, written in permanent ink and the answers added later.

Coloured acetate sheets in yellow, red, blue or green are obtainable, but are more expensive than the ordinary transparent sheet. They can be used for stimulus variation and they do reduce glare. Cellofilm (cellophane in rolls) is disposable and relatively cheap. The rolls are used on the roller bars fitted to the projector. If you are preparing a lecture on the roll, care must be taken to ensure that the ink is dry before winding on, or else the result will be disastrous. Heat from the projector will dry up ink in the pens more quickly than with preparation on the film beforehand. Make sure the tops are replaced on the pens immediately after use.

Acetate marked in differing scales for graphs, shorthand and music are also available. The graph paper is useful for the teaching of electrocardiograms.

Professionally finished coloured transparencies can be made using Transpaseal, which is adhesive on one side. Cut the approximate size to be covered, take off the backing and stick over the area, removing any air bubbles. Using a scalpel, cut off the surplus Transpaseal, without cutting through the base acetate.

Projector Letraset comes in red, blue, green and brown. The letters are transferred clearly.

Film loops, films and video tapes. Motion film can be more readily understood by the use of editing, decreasing the rate of the film and exploding motion sequences. Difficult ideas can be made easier by the use of animation. Movement compels attention, and the use of colour and sound heightens reality. Photography via the microscope enables everyone to see the same view, and minute movements, e.g. phagocytosis of a bacterium by a white blood cell can be seen in motion and therefore be more easily remembered.

Films can be used to influence attitudes, as can video tapes, to an even greater degree. Ward management techniques, human relationship skills, teaching skills and behaviour patterns can be filmed and played back to the group. Discussion can follow about how these could be modified or improved. For instance, could staff and equipment have been used more effectively? Could the approach to the patient have been modified? Did the nurse show

understanding of the patients' needs? Care must be taken to introduce video tape technique gradually, as the experience can be traumatic for most people in the first instance. In time, however,
learners and trained staff welcome the opportunity to see themselves as others see them, and endeavour to improve their skills.

Film loops or mini-films are usually single concept films of a
short length, say ten minutes. Used as an integral part of teaching
they lend themselves to workshops and multi-media situations.
Information is provided by the loop in cassette form. If repeated
showing is desired, this is possible until the idea is fully understood. Revision can be assisted by the use of loops. In nursing
libraries a set of film loops of practical procedures can be made
available, either for revision or to illustrate procedures that have
not been available during a period of ward experience.

When one uses films for teaching, it is important that the teacher
is fully aware of the films that are available. Costs can be reduced
if films are supplied under contract for a set number each month.

Teachers can improve their own demonstration techniques by
observing methods shown in films. Learners can evaluate a film not
only for the content, but also for the teaching method. The
environment in which a film is shown is important. Everyone must
be able to see and hear, and the seating must also be comfortable.
Ventilation is vital to prevent microsleeps!

All teachers must be acquainted with the use of cine projectors.
Before the class the projector must be set up, seating arranged, and
the screen put in place. Make sure that black-out arrangements are
available in the room. Preview of the film is also important as questions posed before the film can aid attention and motivation.
Discussion of the film afterwards can aid the teacher in evaluating
the effectiveness of the film.

Uses of film. Research has shown that people learn from films and
remember sequences. Motivation is heightened, factual knowledge
increased, and opinions may be modified. Careful selection of films
therefore aids learning.

Films used alongside other learning methods add stimulus
variation, and motivate the learner. This function is vital in student
centred learning. There must be an adequate basis of previous
knowledge for learning to take place. The film should reinforce
existing knowledge and then introduce further topics, concepts and
principles. In this way, the learners are encouraged to extend their
knowledge and skills.

Programmed instruction

Many schools of nursing today have teaching machines and books designed for programmed instruction. The material to be learned is logically structured to achieve the presented objectives. Programmed instruction allows the learner to set his own pace, and proceed to the next block of work only when the previous block has been fully mastered.

Many teachers try to compile their own programmed texts, but it must be said that this takes a great deal of time to prepare. Setting precise objectives is important. There are five main steps when compiling a text:

1. State the behavioural objectives to be reached at the end of the programme, i.e. what the learner is expected to be able to *do*.
2. Divide the material into planned blocks in order to achieve the objectives.
3. Break down each block into discrete units of knowledge.
4. Frame questions within each unit to test assimilation. In each step the information has to be provided. Ask pertinent questions or make statements in which the learner fills in the missing words, so that the student's understanding can be tested. There must not be any ambiguous steps in the sequence, since the understanding of each step must facilitate the learning of the next step.
5. Evaluate. Try out the programme on a sample of appropriate students to test the reliability of the sequence. It is important to determine, by a pre-test, the students' background knowledge. A post-test will disclose what the student has learnt from the programme, and whether the objectives have been met.

Each time a teacher prepares a lesson, it should be put into logical sequence, and the preparation of a programmed text is an extension of this activity.

Programmes can be designed to provide comprehensive teaching, drawing on all nursing-related disciplines. This type of sequence could be used to build up a picture of a patient suffering from a specific condition. The programme would include the prerequisite knowledge for understanding the principles and concepts of the pathological process, the development of the abnormal body function and the skills required to nurse the patients and assess their short and long term needs. An outline history of the patient can be given to the learner including his socio-economic background and his emotional response to his illness. By carefully sequencing the programme, the structure and function can be related to the signs and symptoms. The nurse assesses the patient's needs and plans the care to meet the needs.

Programmed texts cannot replace the teacher, but do enable her to give more individual assistance to learners. This involves time, which is a resource requiring careful planning. By relieving the teacher of a heavy load of formal teaching sessions, time is released to assist learners in small groups or individually. In turn, the teacher keeps herself up to date and maintains an *active* interest in motivating and guiding the learner.

Audio-aids

The spoken word is one of the most persuasive and common methods of communication, and remains so, despite the advent of television.

Hearing is one of the senses essential for communication, but it is very often the *use* of the spoken word which presents difficulty in understanding communication. We do not always say what we mean to say, and leave ourselves open to misinterpretation. This is particularly true of people with differing cultures and also of people under stress. Nurses frequently have difficulty in conveying the exact meaning of messages to patients and relatives. Because this skill is vital to a nurse, it must be developed by clinical teachers, tutors and the ward team. Intonation is important. The alteration of stress on certain words can completely change the meaning of a phrase or sentence. In order to reinforce verbal communication, we also use non-verbal communication, such as gestures, posture or facial expressions, and these also need to be discussed.

Critical listening enables nurses to evaluate communication and this skill can be developed by using the radio and teacher-produced tape recordings. A way of improving communications is to assist the learner to become sensitive to the sharing of ideas, discussion of topics and experiences.

The spoken word must be heard clearly. We have all heard of the party game where a message is whispered form one person to the next: 'Send up reinforcements, we are going to advance'. The message at the other end has been distorted to produce send three and fourpence, he is going to a dance'. If we speak, we must also listen, and tape-recording is a good technique for evaluating our own communications.

Listening to fellow colleagues, patients and relatives is an important skill, but we should also teach nurses to be aware of what the patient or relative does *not* say. Is the apparently over-confident patient too afraid to ask a direct question? Is the implication of the answer something that he cannot cope with? How does the nurse cope with these situations? Hard and fast rules cannot be laid down as each individual situation varies, but if nurses participate in discussion and role play, it can help them to have more confidence when they experience the real situation. They can learn from their mistakes at no cost to the relative or the patient. To communicate effectively is an art which also presupposes the ability to listen.

In the teaching of the principles of group discussion, every member of the group should take turns in leading the discussion. As the group becomes more experienced in discussion techniques, its self-confidence should increase. Teachers leading discussions should ask the following questions:

1. Does the attitude of the group facilitate discussion? If not, why not?
2. Has the teacher provided an environment where listening is possible?
3. Has everyone been encouraged or allowed to speak?
4. Are the students encouraged to express their own ideas in discussion?
5. Are the students able to be constructive – not destructive?
6. Are the group members flexible enough to accept ideas and opinions different from their own?

Patients and relatives can be brought into the classroom either in person, or in the form of a taped interview or talk. A possible example of this might be their experiences of bereavement, pre/post-operative preparation, admission/discharge experiences.

Lectures may be recorded on to cassettes for ward or school teaching programmes. Such recordings are useful if made available to learners for revision or to those who have missed the lecture. Trained staff too might find recorded items valuable for their own continuing education.

The recognition of particular sounds has importance in nursing education. Below is a list of sounds which could be useful to reinforce the spoken word:

1. Systolic and diastolic pressure sounds
2. Heart sounds
3. Respirations
   a. obstructive airway disease
   b. Cheyne-Stokes respirations
4. Bowel sounds – normal and abnormal
5. Pleural and pericardial friction rubs
6. Deaf aid simulations
7. Alarm signals
   a. Fire
   b. Monitoring equipment
8. Fire extinguisher release
9. Oxygen valve blow-out
10. Ward noises (night and day)
11. Music used in psychiatry and during childbirth

Rationale for using sound aid:

1. Increases retention of information
2. Increases motivation of the learner
3. Stimulates verbal discussion
4. Demonstrates sound relationships

Workshops

In my introduction to this chapter and throughout its length, I have stressed the importance of the activity of the learner with the teacher acting as facilitator and co-ordinator. A shop is where activity or industry is apparent, where items are sold. Therefore, a workshop in the context of education is envisaged as a place where ideas are exchanged and new concepts and principles are introduced so that they can be discussed, accepted, or rejected by thinking learners. The teacher has items for sale, and whether the learner buys will depend on her:

1. Display of the goods.
2. Encouraging the learner to see a need for the goods.
3. Motivating the learner to buy the goods and use them to the best advantage.

In the workshop, theory and practice are more easily linked by displaying and making available material and practical work, side by side, each depending upon the other for full understanding.

Answers to such questions as:

1. Why does it happen?
2. How does it work?
3. What is it for?

are provided by a range of resources available to the learner, permitting her to find her own answers. Nowhere in a workshop is there room for the learner who wants to sit back and be spoon-fed with facts. Good nursing hinges on the ability to assess, plan, provide and evaluate care for the patient in a given set of circumstances. In other words, we must motivate our learner to think, and give her ample opportunity to do so.

Careful planning, co-ordination and evaluation of workshops are a must. Unless the learner is given careful guidance in using such resources effectively, the whole process is a waste of time for all concerned. How often do you hear learners complain 'What on earth are we expected to do?' or 'How do we go about it?'

Planning a workshop. Firstly, a workshop must have a central theme. This could be an aspect of patient care, such as the prevention of pressure sores, a comprehensive study of a specific health problem such as alcoholism, the problems resulting from a pathological process (e.g. atherosclerosis) or a study of homeostatic mechanisms. Alternatively, the title could be 'Care of the patient suffering from _____' or, 'having difficulty with _____ _____'.

When planning a workshop:

1. Write down your aims and broad objectives.
2. Set your behavioural objectives. Ask what do I expect the nurses to do at the end of the workshop.
3. Assess the facilities that are available. Will you require one large room for the entire week, with subsidiary rooms for practical classes, formal lectures etc., or is one room sufficient? What equipment will be necessary.
4. Find out whether library facilities are available to nurses after 5 p.m. If not, can the workshop be available to the learners and be manned by teaching staff after 5 p.m.? This last factor will depend on the number of teaching staff in the school and working relationships within the department.
5. Decide whether there are any linked educational visits e.g. visits to the community – homes of patients, clinics, health centres,

prisons, factories, museums, schools – can provide a wider perspective than just looking at a topic from the hospital angle.
6. Find out the learners' initial state of knowledge. If they are beginning their training, what is their educational background?

Having decided on your broad aims and objectives and any outside resources which may be required, you should then break these down into the knowledge and skills the nurse requires in order to complete the project.

Next, time-table the programme and identify the formal teaching sessions required to give the learners a firm basis on which to build. This requires an awareness of their present state of knowledge. Link up the theory and practical sessions into a meaningful and logical sequence, allowing time for individual study or small group work.

Decide what teaching resources you will need for the formal teaching sessions. These sessions should be reinforced using the resources in the workshop and in the classes on clinical nursing care. The overall design of the workshop will depend on structural facilities of the school and also the number of willing teaching staff. One tutor or clinical teacher would find it impossible to work in isolation. A team effort is required. The pooling of resources, personalities and skills is essential for a forward-looking approach to education. Furthermore, learners very often find a team approach to patient care productive since the caring team are seen, *as a team*, linking hospital and community services.

From the objectives a workbook must be planned. Each learner should have a copy of the objectives. A reading list must be compiled. The librarian may be able to assist you with this, and also any tape-slide presentations or video tapes. You may be able to have these resources in the workshop to enable group viewing if the number of students is large.

The design of the area will depend upon whether you have a practical room available (dissection, if you are including this, will require hand washing facilities), a reading area and somewhere for the provision of supplementary reading, and whether the library can be used.

Further resources

Models. These are for the learner to *use*, to handle, take apart and put together again. The student should identify the specific parts and relate the structure to the function. Real specimens too can be available so that the size of an organ, or the appearance of tissue can be appreciated.

Dissection of animal organs aids in the reinforcement of lectures – e.g. an ox heart, lambs' kidneys etc. Instructions on how to dissect the organ must be given and guidance as to the parts the learner is to identify, draw, describe etc., based on the objectives.

Displays to illustrate important points. Here, the use of charts, either commercially produced or designed by the teaching staff, are useful. Nursing procedures can be shown effectively in display form, e.g. urinary drainage – what are the underlying principles involved? What instructions must be given to nurses caring for the patient? What special needs does the patient have if catheter drainage is implemented? There are many aspects which can be considered using this layout. Flip charts can be used either to give information, to describe a sequence of events, or to ask more searching questions for discussion later.

Dietetic treatments form an important part of treatment in some cases. A display depicting the abnormal function, the dietetic correction and the principles involved, plus a display of foods available, can, with imagination, be depicted in visual form.

Co-ordination of the workshop

In order that the learner uses the workshop to the best advantage, a full introductory explanation must be given. To some learners it may be a completely new experience. Discussion should take place regarding the learning methods, i.e. practical work, discussions, role play, tutorials and individual study.

The workbook should be distributed at the beginning of the week/day, together with the aims and objectives for the shop. If the workshop is planned to accompany a module of nursing experience, the ward *and* school objectives can be given so that the learner comes to see the ward and school staff as a complete team. The workbook can include questions to answer, observations to make, care plans to complete and topics for essays to be written. Reading lists including relevant research and articles from journals should be appended.

The learning that is expected from the accompanying ward experience can be made explicit, and here the names of the staff who might act as resource personnel can help the new learner particularly. Projects (or nursing care studies) could be suggested to complete in the ward situation. Studies that reach a high standard can be submittted for publication.

Last but by no means least, the book should include the learner's own evaluation of the workshop and a final evaluation of the complete learning module, both in the school and the ward.

How to use the workshop

Each learner should be assigned to a clinical teacher or tutor whom they should consult regarding individual difficulties. The same teacher should also be responsible for group tutorials. Teachers should be active when in the shop and approach the learners; sometimes the learner holds back because she feels she is the only one with difficulties. The teacher can get together a small group to discuss problems. In this way, each student gets individualised assistance according to her special needs.

Worksheets and hand-outs

What is the difference between a worksheet and a handout? Sometimes it is difficult to separate the two, but basically a hand-out is a prepared statement complete in itself, whereas, a worksheet requires student effort to complete and should stimulate further work.

Hand-outs. Learners like hand-outs, but they should not be used with monotonous regularity to echo everything the teacher says. If this is the case, they will not be used by the student. Hand-outs usually give information and therefore the information must be accurate and set out in such a way that it can be easily read and understood. Difficult concepts can be illustrated on a hand-out as diagrams or graphs, backed up by short, clear, written statements. The hand-out can be given out at the beginning of the learning session and used as a basis for teaching. This ensures that each learner has a chance in class to go through the handout and study it. The sheet can be retained for revision purposes. The device ensures that the students have the correct information and avoids copious note-taking.

Hand-outs can also be given at the end of the teaching session or sequence. For instance, to summarise small group work or seminars. The information produced can be amalgamated and distributed to all the learners, so that everyone has the benefit of the work of the entire group. At the end of a lesson, a hand-out can summarise important points thus allowing full concentration and attention during the instruction.

I have already mentioned some information that can be included on a hand-out, e.g. reading lists, training plans, aims and objectives.

Diagrams, graphs, etc. may also be given as hand-outs. Before preparing any hand-out, however, teachers must ask themselves *why* they are giving it and how they are to use it. – Is it to be used in class, or as an evaluation tool? Is it an objective that the learner be able to draw the particular diagram? If so, would it be better if they reproduced it themselves? Is it to be given to ensure that everyone has the correct drawing or to save time? A diagram may be used to summarise a lecture, or group of lectures, or to outline a plan. Any drawing must be large enough to be clearly seen and also set the standard for items produced by the learner.

Worksheets. These provide a basis for further instruction, either with the assistance of the teacher, or for individual work. Care must be taken to ensure that completed worksheets are evaluated.

A worksheet can be used as a preparation for role play. Situations and characters to be portrayed can be set out for the learner on a worksheet. Each student receives different instructions and this allows for spontaneity of reactions, thus making the situation more real.

Worksheets can provide feedback for the teacher. They can be distributed at the completion of the teaching and worked through under test conditions, e.g. multiple choice, true false questions. They can also be used to evaluate the teacher, when they might include questions such as:

1. Do the students feel the teacher has enabled them to achieve the objectives?
2. Was all of the teaching clear?
3. Could the topic perhaps be put in a different way?
4. Should anything else be included/excluded, stating the reasons why?
5. Which aspects of the learning experience have been most enjoyable and why?
6. Were the visits useful?

Whether it is a hand-out or a worksheet, a critical look is important. One should consider the following:

1. Does the hand-out/worksheet do what it is meant to do?
2. Are the questions clear and unambiguous?

3. If it is a test, is it valid? Does it test what it sets out to test?
4. Are the questions reliable?
5. Is the information given up to date? Should any additional references be included?
6. Does the hand-out need revising in the light of new reports etc?
7. Is the document motivating in its content and presentation?
8. Does it assist the learner to be creative and outward-looking in her work?

In conclusion, when considering the inclusion of any teaching resource in one's teaching programme, one should bear in mind that:

> The whole art of teaching is only the art of awakening the natural curiosity of young minds for the purpose of satisfying it afterwards.
>
> *Anatole France.*

COMPANIES FOR FILM HIRE ETC.

Abbott Laboratories, Queensborough, Kent ME11 SE11
Ames Co. (Miles Laboratories), Stoke Poges, Slough SL24 2L
Armour Pharmaceuticals Co. Ltd, Hampden Park, Eastbourne, Sussex BN22 9AG
Ayerst Laboratories Ltd., Invincible Road, Farnborough, Hants GU14 7QH
Beecham Research Laboratories, Beecham House, Brentford, Middlesex
Boehringer Ingleheim Ltd, Southern Industrial Estate, Bracknell, Berkshire RG12 4YS
CIBA Laboratories, Dudley House, High Street, Cranleigh, Surrey GU6 8AE
Cow and Gate, Trowbridge, PO Box 99, Wiltshire
Eaton Laboratories, Regent House, The Broadway, Woking, Surrey GU21 5AP
Farley Health Products, Torr Lane, Plymouth, Devon PL3 5AU
Fisons Ltd Pharmaceutical Division, 12 Derby Road, Loughbourough, Leicestershire
Glaxo Laboratories Ltd, Greenford, Middlesex
Heinz Cookery Service, Hayes Park, Hayes, Middlesex
Hoechst (UK) Ltd Pharmaceutical Division, Hoechst House, Salisbury, Wiltshire, TW4 6JH
Kabi Vitrum Ltd, Bilton House, Uxbridge Road, Ealing Monoject Division, Sherwood Medical Ltd, London Road, County Oak, Crawley, W. Sussex
Pharmax Ltd, Bourne Road, Bexley, Kent DA51 NX
Reckitt & Colman (Pharmaceutical Division), Dansom Lane, Hull
Riker Laboratories (3M's Laboratory Ltd), 1 Morley Street, Loughborough, Leicester LE11 1EP
Roussell Nutrition Division, Roussell House, Wembley Park, Wembley, Middlesex HAG ONF
Travenol Laboratories Ltd, Caxton Way, Thetford, Norfolk IP24 35E
Searle Laboratories, PO Box 53, Lane End Road, High Wycombe, Bucks HP12 4HL

Seton, Tubiton House, Medlock Street, Oldham OL1 345
Winthrope Laboratories, Sterling-Winthrope House, Surbiton-on-Thames, Surrey KT6 4PH

USEFUL ADDRESSES

Age Concern, 60 Pitcairn Road, Mitcham, Surrey CR4 3LL
Bailliere Tindall, 1 Vincent Square, London SW1P 2PN
Banda Visual Aids, NIG Banda Ltd, Colchester, Essex CO1 1XU
BBC Publications, PO Box 234, London SE1 3TH
British Diabetic Association, 3–6 Alfred Place, London WC1E 7EE
Camera Talks Ltd, 31 North Row, London W1
Catalogue of Dental Health Education Material, General Dental Council, 37 Wimpole Street, London W1 M 8DQ
Central Film Library, Chalfont Grove, Narcot Lane, Gerrards Cross, Bucks SL9 8TN
Coeliac Society, PO Box 181, London NW2 2QY
Concorde Films Council, 201 Felixstowe Road, Ipswich, Suffolk 1P3 9BF
Council for Educational Technology, 3 Devonshire Street, London WIN 2BA
Cystic Fibrosis Society, 5 Blyth Road, Bromley, Kent BR1 3RS
Disabled Living Foundation, 346 Kensington High Street, London W14 8NS
Graves Medical Audio-visual Library, Holly House, 220 New London Road, Chelmsford CM2 9BJ
Guild of Sound and Vision Ltd, Woodston House, 85–129 Oundle Road, Peterborough PE2 9PZ
Health Education Council, 78 New Oxford Street, London WC1A LAH
Help The Aged Education Department, 218 Upper Street, London N1
Mavis Medical Audio-visual Information Service, University of Dundee, Ninewells Hospital, Dundee DD1 95Y
Medical Recording Foundation, PO Box 99, Chelmsford CM1 5HL
Multiple Sclerosis Society, 286 Munster Road, London SW6
National Audio-visual Aids Centre, Paxton Place, London SE27
NHS Learning Resources Unit, 55 Broomgrove Road, Sheffield S10 2NA
Oxford Educational Resources (AVNT), 197 Batley Road, Oxford OX2 OHE
Royal National Institute for the Blind, 224–6–8 Great Portland Street, London WIN 6AA
Royal National Institute for the Deaf, Gower Street, London WC1
TALC Foundation for teaching aids at low cost, PO Box 49, St Albans, Herts AL1 4AX
Teaching aids at low cost, Institute of Child Health, 30 Guildford Street, London WC1
Smith & Nephew Medical Film Library, 15 Beaconsfield Road, London NW10 2LE
Wellcome Foundation Ltd, Wellcome Institute, 183 Euston Road, London NW1 2BP

REFERENCES

Allen, M. A. (1981) Production of a video tape. *Nursing times*, May 21st, 915–916.
Ashworth, P. (1980) *Care to Communicate*. London: Royal College of Nursing.
Bendall, E. (1976) Teaching for reality. *Journal of Advanced Nursing*, 1, 3–9.
Boreham, N. C. (1977) Use of case histories to assess nurses' ability to solve clinical problems. *Journal of Advanced Nursing Studies*, 2, 57–66.

Cable, R. (1972) *Audio Visual Aid Handbook*. London: University of London Press.

Clamp, C. (1980) Learning through incidents. *Nursing Times*, **76**, 1755–1758.

Coleman, Violet A. (1973) Teaching in a specialised unit. *Nursing Times*, June 21.

Coppen, Helen (1964) *Wall Sheets, Their Designs, Production and use*. London: National Council for Audio-visual aids.

Coppen, Helen (1969) *Aids to Teaching and Learning* Oxford: Pergamon Press.

Dale, E. (1969) *Audio-visual Methods in Teaching*, 3rd edn. New York: Holt, Rinehart and Winston.

Dolgarno, J. (1977) The audio visual aids technician. *Nursing Times*, April 21.

Eric, E. D. (1977) Achievement gains in multi media instruction and conventional lecture methods. Virginia, U.S.A.

Faulkner, A. (1981) Communication skills. *Nursing Times*, **77**, 332–6.

French, P. (1980) Academic gaming in nurse education. *Journal of Advanced Nursing*, No. 6, 601–612.

Hewton, E. & Holder, M. (1973) A school resources centre. *British Journal of Educational Technology*, No.1 **4**, 41–53.

Jones, W. J. (1981) Self-directed learning. *Journal of Advanced Nursing*, No. 6, 59–69.

Kataoka, Winifred (1966) How to develop an audio visual aid bank. *Nursing Outlook*, No. 14, 49–50.

Kinder, James S. (1965) *Using Audio-visual Materials in Education*. New York: American Book Co.

Marson, S. N. (1976) Educational technology. A moment for change. *Journal of Advanced Nursing*, No.2, **1**, 155–162.

Marson, S. N. (1977) Nursing Education and Educational Technology. *Nursing Times*, April 21.

McLelean, S. R. (1973) *Ready for Report, Nurse?* London: Royal College of Nursing.

MacMillan, P. (1981) Communication skills. *Nursing Times*, **77**, 151–152 and 354–5.

National Council for Audio Visual Aids (1965) *Guide for the Production of Wall-charts*.

Neame, R. L. B. (1981) How to construct a problem-based course. *Medical Teacher*, **3**, No. 3.

Perry, E. (1981) Communication. Series 1–4. *Nursing Mirror*, 152, 22–3; 24–6; 26–8; 34–5.

Robinson, Geraldine (1966) How to develop an Audio visual aid bank. *Nursing Outlook*, No. 14, 49–50.

Stephen, Shirley (1977) Audio-visual aids and the libraries' role. *Nursing Times*, April 21.

Tabor, R. B. (1977) Libraries and information for nurses. *Nursing Times*, March 11.

Townsend, Ian (1976) Educational technology. A moment for change. *Journal of Advanced Nursing*, No.2, **1**, 155–162.

Townsend, Ian (1977) A Utopian view of the centre and its role in the nurse training school. *Nursing Times*, April 14.

Townsend, Ian (1977) Results of Surveys by the National Health Service Learning Resources Unit. *Nursing Times*, May 19.

Townsend, Ian (1977) Using Audio-visual equipment. *Nursing Times*, June 10.

University of Exeter (1971) Visual Communication in Engineering Science. *British Journal of Educational Technology No. 1*. **2**, January.

Warwick, David. *Team Teaching*. University of London Press Ltd.

Wilkes, John. *Under-utilisation of Audio-visual Aids*. New University of Ulster, Coleraine, N. Ireland.

Wittich & Schuler. *Audio-visual Materials*. 4th Edition. Harper & Row.

7

Teaching psychiatric nursing in the clinical situation

Psychiatric nurses sometimes use skills which involve manual dexterity and the use of technical equipment, and the teaching of such skills is recorded elsewhere in this book.

This chapter will concentrate on other nursing skills which have particular significance in psychiatric care. These are:

1. Observation skills
2. Communication skills
3. Human relationship skills

With increased recognition of the need to plan and deliver care suitable to each individual patient, the importance of these skills for all nurses becomes obvious.

However, particular problems exist in all three areas of skill in psychiatric nursing because of the distortions of perception, thought and behaviour which underlie some disorders.

The new Syllabus introduced in 1982 for courses leading to registration as a mental nurse (unfortunately the old legal terminology remains) is based on the need of the nurse to respond to the behaviour of those being cared for. The skills considered in this chapter are part of the repertoire to enable such responses.

Each group of skills will be discussed separately, to achieve clarity, but it must be recognised that there are no rigid divisions; for example, in order to report or share observations, communication skills are necessary, and communications are enhanced if relationships with others are good.

Observation skills

Much observation in daily life takes place without conscious effort, and the knowledge gained is used in ways which do not seem to require conscious planning. An example would be a slight lengthening of stride to avoid a small puddle after rain.

151

So many stimuli bombard the senses, that only those which seem to have significance can be selected for attention. The walker mentioned above, avoiding the puddle, was probably even less aware of similar hazards on the other side of the street, as they did not lie on his route.

Selection of appropriate stimuli, and use of the information in a helpful manner, is developed with experience so that it takes place without conscious effort, in order that normal activities can be facilitated. However, in observing unusual phenomena, a conscious, systematic approach must be fostered in the nurse learner. Skill in observation includes:

1. Careful, systematic use of senses
2. Consideration of the sensory inputs in the situation in which they occur
3. Utilisation of the new information in the light of clinical knowledge and experience
4. Verbalising the observations and interpretations

A person might be observed to be crying; if she is also seen to be peeling onions, no further action is likely to be needed. If, however, there is no obvious cause to be found, further information is needed before interpretation of the event can be undertaken with any certainty.

To foster systematic observation in nurse learners, good use can be made of any clinical situation in which she happens to be working.

After a discussion about the subject of perception, including attention and selection of those features which seem important, it is useful to focus on the static aspects of the environment. These are easily checked by the teacher, and have the additional advantage of remaining the same so that they can be re-assessed by the learner. For example, the number and situation of doors and windows are constant features, and while accompanying patients from room to room, or adjusting ventilation, attention can be drawn to, e.g. width of doorways, designated fire doors, types of glass, e.g. in bathroom windows. An appreciation of such features of patients' living conditions are a prelude to improving comfort, e.g. by avoiding draughty areas in the winter and preserving modesty by drawing curtains over unprotected windows. Mobile aspects of living areas can be focussed on next, e.g. grouping of chairs in relation to windows with views, or the television set, or dining tables. Conscious efforts to notice furniture arrangements will make the nurse more aware of possibilities for adjustment to meet the needs of individuals.

Having introduced the topic of observation by emphasising the importance of relatively stable elements of the patient area, I turn to observation of features of human behaviour, in relation to that environment. 'Observing' a person is much more complex than observing other features of the environment. Behaviour is not static, and although behaviour patterns may emerge, they do not remain constant under all circumstances. The behaviour of an individual is often seen to be modified in the presence of others, and observation itself may influence behaviour.

It is possible to help the nurse to observe behaviour in a clinical setting by:

1. Ensuring that she is able to use her powers of observation in non-clinical situations, and
2. By giving guidance on features of behaviour which may be observed.

People all produce some kind of 'behaviour', so any situation involving people provides adequate teaching and learning opportunities.

One way of showing a nurse what is involved in observing people is to begin with one feature, e.g. dress, which is constant in most clinical and non-clinical situations.

She could be asked to describe the clothes of the person who was last to leave the room. The description would then be compared with notes made previously by the teacher, or the actual clothes, if the individual were still in the vicinity. This exercise can be repeated until the learner's attention to the clothes worn by people in her environment is improved. During this time, she will become more aware of individual styles of dress, and will be able to use clothes as one factor in describing behaviour.

For example, the uniform worn by the ward sister may differ from those of the student nurse, to denote difference in status. The clothes worn by elderly ladies will usually show differences from those worn by teenage girls. A person may well adopt differing styles of clothing depending on the situation, e.g. smart suit for interview, jeans and sweater for relaxing.

From observing the social significance of clothes, progress can be made to observing the dress of those in the clinical situation. Here, social norms may not always govern dress and factors important to the individual may have great influence.

Having had experience of observing one aspect of human behaviour, the learner can progress further. Progression may depend to some extent on the clinical environment.

If the nurse has responsibility for the care of only one or two patients, further individual features of behaviour would be observed. These could include, e.g. facial expression, gait, posture.

If the nurse has a part to play in the care of a large number of patients, the study of aspects of group behaviour could be a more appropriate step.

In early stages it is important that the teacher gives guidance on what, and how, to observe. The learner may have had introductory classes on features of individual and group behaviour; if not, she will need a tutorial on the subject in order to enhance her understanding of what is observed.

If she is observing the behaviour of a group of people, she needs to be aware of the potential for influence of the individual on the group, and of the group on the individual. She may note that one member reluctantly agrees to fit in with the plans of the others, and this may encourage her to look for signs of approval of his action which would make his acquiescence seem worthwhile.

If a group member fails to comply with a majority decision, she will be able to note the behaviour of individuals in the context of possible group pressure. This gives coherence and form to the observations, but rigidity must be avoided by frequently checking that all relevant behaviour has been taken into account.

Some students are helped by having a written scheme of observation to which to work. The teacher in any given clinical situation can devise a suitable scheme.

A scheme for observing individual behaviour would include such items as:

1. Time of day
2. Other people involved
3. Gait
4. Posture
5. Gaze
6. Mannerisms
7. Relationships with others

A very comprehensive list of possible observations can be drawn up, and some learners and teachers feel more confident with this kind of written guideline.

The observations would take place during any activities in which the nurse and patient would normally be involved, and the chart completed at some convenient time later in the day. Experience with such a scheme will be useful to the nurse when she is involved later with assessing patients' levels of competence and progress.

Observations themselves of course do not stand alone. It has already been said that the nurse is more able to observe important features if relevant psychological theory is applied. Clinical knowledge will increase with experience, and this knowledge can also be applied in the process of 'observation'.

If a depressed patient's motor retardation seemed lessened since his treatment by electroplexy began, the nurse who understands the implications will be alert in her observations for signs of suicidal intent, as well as for the more welcome signs such as a greater measure of competence in daily living activities.

Discussion of the observations made, and their significance with experienced personnel are of great value to the learner. She will have feedback on the accuracy of her observations, and of their significance in that particular setting.

She will gain concepts of the ways in which mental disorders affect overt behaviour; but at the same time be able to appreciate the influence the personality of the individual has on the behaviour shown. The experienced nurse will be able to help the nurse learner to avoid the pitfall of stereotyping. By emphasising individual differences which occur in the behaviour of people with the same diagnosis, the teacher can guide the learner into good psychiatric nursing practice.

It is possible to be concerned with only those aspects of observed behaviour which give support to a diagnosis. However, much greater value accrues to the patient if the nurse is equally concerned with his unique features, or the features of normal social behaviour which are retained.

When desired behaviour is reinforced, instead of undesirable or abnormal behaviour, the patient's own strengths are being used to enhance his social competence. If, however, only disordered behaviour seems to be of interest to the staff, his social competence will diminish as his abnormal behaviour increases.

Before leaving the learner to increase her experience in observation, she will need to be aware of the influence of an observer on what is being observed.

She may be able to produce examples from her own life – e.g. how she dresses for different occasions, how she would sit and watch a film in a cinema, or alone watching television, how she would act to attract someone she was interested in, or to give an opposite message to someone she was not interested in! Many behavioural changes are more subtle and will be mentioned again in the section on inter-personal relationships.

It is important that an observer knows that there are constraints upon what she gains from the environment.

Psychological theory explains that the perception of the individual is unique, and involves selecting stimuli in accordance with past experiences and present needs. This, of course, means that some potential inputs are ignored.

The stimuli, once selected, are then processed and distortions can take place, and most learners will be able to contribute ideas.

For example, people can be viewed as

1. The idle gossip, or interesting conversationalist
2. The foolhardy risk taker, or brave explorer
3. The generous person, or spendthrift

These examples are of extremes, and there are many opportunities for distortion between the extreme end points.

Attitudes and prejudices distort perception. Current personal needs influence selection of stimuli. Expectations of a situation may also have great bearing on the information gleaned from observation of that situation.

As her experience in observation grows, the learner will be able to utilise psychological theory in her thinking about patients and their situations. The teacher can encourage her to co-ordinate theoretical knowledge with practical work by working with the learner to examine her reported observations, and the conclusions drawn. Alternative conclusions can be discussed, with reasons for discarding these, and the reported observations can be compared (for example) with those of another learner, to see where and how perceptions of a situation differed.

Learners can help each other when a teacher is not available, by acting as checks for each other's observations.

Observations can be used in writing nurses' notes for those patients in the care of a particular learner, and experience can be gained in articulating what has been observed in ward meetings, and any therapeutic groups in which the nurse may participate.

The methodical approach to observing and describing events which has been discussed above is helpful when a nurse has the opportunity to make some contribution in a meeting.

'Mrs Smith was rather depressed this morning' is certainly vague when compared with a recounting of behavioural changes noted, e.g. failure to respond to morning greetings, reluctance to go to wash, request to go without breakfast, and have a cup of tea away from the table, effort to isolate herself by sitting in a normally little used part of the sitting room.

The fuller communication of Mrs Smith's behaviour gives specific pointers to the nursing care she will need, and (as was said at the beginning of the chapter) careful observation is a prerequisite for the planning of individual care. She will need some help with skin and mouth care, and further investigations are needed about food. She may prefer fluids for the day, in which case something more nutritious than tea will be offered. If she wants to eat at lunch time it may be best to arrange for her to eat alone, if she is still avoiding other people. Above all, it is obvious that she needs time – time to respond to conversation, time to be cared for separately rather than in a group, time to relate to one individual rather than a team of staff.

The learner needs to know that her work has value, and when her observations are sufficiently detailed, careful and relevant to be used as a basis for discussion and planning care, her efforts will be rewarded.

Once a care plan is formulated, it is necessary to assess the validity at intervals, especially whenever nursing intervention has taken place. The teacher can reinforce the value of accurate observation by showing the learner how to use her findings to assess the success of a nursing intervention.

Skills only have value if purpose can be shown. It has been known for nurses' notes to be kept but not utilised. It is important for nurses to recognise the value of nursing observations, and to use the findings themselves. Nursing care must be devised and directed by nurses, and well presented observations form a sound basis for the nursing process.

Summary

1. Observations in daily life are often made and utilised at subconscious levels.
2. Observations in the clinical area for the nurse learner must be facilitated by bringing aspects of the environment to conscious notice.

3. Observations of static aspects of the environment (e.g. building) are useful starting points.
4. They are easily checked, and awareness of these aspects may enhance nursing care later.
5. Further non-human aspects of the environment can be included when the nurse has shown ability to discuss her observations of the static aspects.
6. Complex human behaviour is not easily observed, so the teacher must simplify the requirements for the nurse learner.
7. The student can initially focus on an aspect of behaviour which is common to clinical and non-clinical situations.
8. When experience has been gained in this aspect, further elements of behaviour can be added.
9. The clinical situation will dictate progression at this point- aspects of individual behaviour can be added if the nurse is involved in the care of only a few patients – aspects of group behaviour would be more appropriate if she is involved in the care of a large number of patients.
10. By allowing the learner to increase her skill in observation in small steps, relevant theoretical inputs can also be introduced at appropriate times.
11. Theories of perception and concept formation can be introduced, showing strengths and weaknesses in relation to observation of human behaviour.
12. Knowledge of psychiatric illness will increase with experience, and this can be utilised in conjunction with observations to build up concepts of disorders, as well as appreciation of the differences shown by individuals suffering from the same disorder.
13. Clinical observations are an essential prelude to the formulation of nursing policy, especially where individual care plans are implemented.

Communication skills

Communications play a large part in human interaction. Communications can be oral, written or nonverbal and the context is important.

During socialisation, individuals learn ways of communicating with each other in various social settings, and everyone within a given culture acquires knowledge of conventions and formalising which facilitate smooth interactions.

Conventions include the phrases used in greetings, and formalities indicate attempts to eliminate ambiguity within a certain context, such as in the standard police caution.

Human communication is varied and sophisticated, as manifested by our refined use of language.

Animals without language have a much more limited range of communication with each other. However, having the ability to use words as symbols has disadvantages too. The range of messages which can be exchanged is great, and the possibilities for misinterpretation are also great.

It is also possible for the verbal message to convey one meaning, while the nonverbal behaviour conveys a different meaning.

In addition to its use in social interaction, language has other functions. Groups of people use language in ways which are specific to the group; this includes the language of the country, such as English of French, and the language of sub-groups such as work groups and drug sub-cultures. The use of language within the group maintains a sense of identity, and transmits the group's history in its own unique way.

Written or spoken words are usually used in deliberate ways, with intention to convey and give messages. The message can be enhanced by nonverbal signals, or (as mentioned above) it can be negated or confused. Much of nonverbal communication is not deliberate, and this is a further complicating factor in human communications.

This brief survey of the factors involved in everyday social communication should indicate the even greater complexity of communicating with people with psychiatric disorders involving thought and speech disorders. It is important that the nurse learner acquires a knowledge of aspects of communication in normal interactions as a basis for understanding the problems in abnormal situations. As communication is part of everyday life, the teacher can use any clinical or classroom situation to help the learner. Some of the important words from the preceding paragraphs could be used as bases for learning.

Oral communications

Students may surprise themselves with how much they know, but do not verbalise, about oral communications.

After three or four weeks of experience as nurse learners, it is useful to ask them to state how their ways of speaking to each other have changed during their time together. Having grown to know each other, and worked together, formality will have been reduced. More time will be spent talking with some people than with others. Topics of conversation will have changed as each member finds others with similar interests and as the whole group gains more shared experiences.

The teacher must help the learners to look for reasons for the changes that are mentioned. For example, shared experiences means that members have a common base of knowledge which can be assumed in future conversations on the topic, eliminating the need for preliminary explanations. This is important, as misunderstandings and confusion can arise if knowledge is mistakenly assumed.

Reduction of formality is a feature of speech among those who know each other well. However, a newcomer to the group may well feel an intruder as his speech will initially be more formal.

It is pleasant to find members of the group who share a common interest; but the disadvantages may be that interests are narrowed because of the specific focus, and that some members of the group may feel excluded. It is important that the teacher helps students to be aware of the positive and negative aspects of the changes mentioned, because this will lead to an understanding of the effects of familiarity, shared knowledge and group interests in other situations.

Early in nursing experience, the special language needed is introduced. Professional terminology is essential so its use is encouraged. There is often also a tendency for another language to emerge, made up of abbreviations and distortions, understood (albeit imperfectly) by those using it, but frequently annoying and confusing to those who do not use it. The story of the student nurse who told the night sister that 'P.P.O.' in the day report meant 'please prepare for operation' and that 'P.P.O.' in the night report meant 'patient prepared for operation' illustrates this point. This kind of language is used to mark a group of people from others, and a very good example is the special and ever-changing vocabulary of drug abusers. Here terms tend to change frequently in order that the initiated are easily recognisable. This has the effect of including only those who show evidence of knowledge, and excluding all others, thus protecting those who are involved in illicit acts from possible infiltration. It may be that with more security in the value of themselves as professional people, nurses will abandon the tendency to use distorted speech forms, and will use professional terminology instead. Tape recorders are useful in drawing the attention of speakers to their use of words. Recordings can be made of classroom discussions or ward discussions and tutorials, and the way in which words were used could be considered afterwards.

Words used should be appropriate in the context. Professional terminology is necessary among those who share experience of such words. One function that a nurse frequently has to perform is to accept a piece of information from one source and express it in different words to enable it to be understood by others. There is a music hall monologue about a person who had been prescribed some medicine to be taken in a recumbent posture. The story tells at length of the search to find a recumbent posture in which to put the medicine. There are, of course, recent parallels for this story, illustrating the need for one of the communication skills of the nurse – to express a message in different words, without losing the original meaning. A useful exercise can be carried out in ward tutorials, or in the classroom. One learner speaks for a short time on a given topic, and a second learner rephrases in her own words. The material can be original, from the first learner's own experience, or it could be sections read from patients' notes, ward reports, instruction cards for patients, text books, or newspaper and journal articles. This is also a useful aid to learning the material being discussed. Following a rephrasing session nurses could be asked to note times in the clinical situation when they became aware of rephrasing, and the reasons for changing the words. Reasons would include:

1. A suspicion that the message would not be understood, or acceptable, in original form.
2. A response to a request for clarification.
3. An attempt to correct a misunderstanding.
4. An effort to save time.
5. To give the message more immediate impact.

The aids to learning mentioned here will enhance the other means of improving knowledge of oral communications which will be used, e.g. practice in reporting in the clinical situation, and increased experience with patients and staff.

Written communications

The spoken word is usually transitory (except when recorded on tape for some reason). The written word is more permanent, and, as such, can be used long after the writer has forgotten the incident, or is no longer in the vicinity. For instance, a patient readmitted after a five year gap may not be known to any of the present staff, so his records should be an accurate summary of his illness and progress.

In addition to patient related notes, the nurse will need to requisition supplies, request services, complete charts and forms, help some patients with correspondence, and, of course, complete her written work in connection with her studies.

Written communications are usually read in the absence of the writer, so clarification cannot easily be sought. It is essential, therefore, that nurse learners have practice in producing concise, accurate information in written form. Some of the exercises already mentioned under the heading 'Observation Skills' will be useful in this context. For example, when a patient's behaviour is being observed, written notes can be made, enabling the nurse to develop both observation and recording skills together.

Reading good reports written by other staff members, and relating these to the patients concerned is one way of learning how to make useful notes.

It is important that a learner knows why she is to write about a patient or a situation. The more important the reason, the more effort can be expected. If nurses' notes are to be used as a basis for assessment of nursing care needs, the learner will know that the overworked word 'comfortable' is not helpful, and that some expression of the events which have made the patient more comfortable would be of reater value. On the other hand, if records are being kept for a single specific purpose, only that information requested should be recorded. For example, if a survey is being made of the incidence of patients wearing dentures, that is the only information of value in that context.

In the clinical environment various forms and charts have been devised in order to simplify and clarify communications between those responsible for patient care. The nurse will need instruction on how to complete such forms, but in order that accuracy is assured, she will need to know why the information is important and how it will be used. As in most learning, early feedback is very rewarding, and when she can see that a patient's care plan is adjusted, taking into account the observations she has made, the nurse learner will have confirmation of the necessity of accuracy in making and in recording observations.

While discussing written communications, whatever the clinical context, the teacher has a good opportunity to include other examples, such as forms giving consent for treatment and patients' prescription cards. Such documents can give information to the nurse, and to others, and their importance can be stressed here.

Many opportunities arise in the classroom for improving written work, and some of these opportunities carry over into the clinical area. For example, care studies can provide a method of helping the nurse to make concise, accurate notes about a patient in her care, for a purpose related to her own education. The notes would include:

1. Records of the nurses' observations and assessment
2. Summaries of the patients' medical history
3. Information from observation charts, care plans etc.

This gives the nurse practice in taking information from a variety of sources and putting it in writing, into her own words, in a way which is useful to the person who is going to read and assess it

While undertaking practice in written communications, it is essential that the learner is given information on acceptable abbreviations which she may use. It is unnecessary to waste time if some abbreviations are permitted (for instance, those relating to quantities of drugs), but it is important to avoid non-standard contractions.

Nonverbal communications

Nonverbal communications are important in human interaction. They include eye gaze, facial expressions, body posture, distance or closeness and gestures.

The nonverbal expressions can enhance or re-inforce a verbal message. A smile, a handshake, and remaining close will encourage a listener to believe the speaker who says he is glad to see him.

A gesture can take the place of a verbal message – pointing to the right can indicate direction in the same way as verbal instruction to take the road to the right.

A further function of nonverbal communication is to give texture to the social setting, that is, it need not be concerned with the actual verbal message being conveyed, but it is concerned with conveying information about aspects of the situation such as interest in the individual, acceptance, approval, or negative aspects such as rejection or boredom.

Much nonverbal activity takes place without the individual being conscious of it, and learners need to identify these activites and to observe what functions are served in different situations.

A great deal of useful observation can be undertaken in everyday situations, to help the learner become more aware of nonverbal activities.

Travellers on public transport in Britain are well known for their avoidance of verbal communication, but a great deal of nonverbal interaction is common. The ways in which personal space is protected are interesting. Shopping bags and brief cases are used to discourage newcomers from sitting too close; eye gaze is avoided; shuffling movements of the feet gain time while a new passenger looks for a seat, but no actual extra space is made for him to sit; these are some examples. It is also useful to note how people arrange themselves and the furniture if they wish to talk to each other for example, in the nurses' sitting room, or a common room. The postures and gestures of those who are deep in conversation can be compared with the physical movements of those who are alone or not in conversation.

Appearance is nonverbal, but can produce a number of signals. Learners could think of the clothes they would wear on different occasions, and why, and they could also discuss the clothes and appearance they would expect from others in different situations, for example, on duty, at a party, for an interview for a new post.

When considering their ideas about clothes and appearance it is appropriate to enable the learners to explore their own attitudes towards people whose appearances do not conform to their own ideas, for example, the person who never appears in casual dress, or the individual who always seems unwashed.

Awareness of nonverbal features of communications in the clinical setting is important and after the general introduction outlined above, the nurse can use her clinical assignments to gain more insight in this area. Eye gaze, facial expressions and gestures are all part of normal communications between staff, and the learner should be encouraged to look for these and see what functions they serve. People who work closely together often reduce the need for explicit word messages because of the significance of the nonverbal messages. Familiarity with a situation enables verbal explanations to be reduced and nonverbal signals may well be substituted for words. This situation could be contrasted with that of a nurse new to the ward who had not got the shared experiences of others to enable her to gain understanding without a great deal of verbal explanation.

Absence of something familiar often shows its true value and if the nurse undertakes the care of a blind patient, she will be aware of the difference the absence of eye gaze and reciprocal facial expressions makes to ease of conversation. Role play can be used, with students closing their eyes to reduce nonverbal cues.

When the nurse is ready to look for nonverbal cues, she will be able to investigate at least some of her own behaviour. In many clinical situations, physical contact takes the place of verbal messages. The confused old lady responds better to a comforting arm around her shoulders and help to hold her teacup, than to kind words of persuasion, which she cannot comprehend.

Although written, oral and nonverbal aspects of communication have been discussed separately, this does not imply that each aspect is totally separate. In addition, the context in which any communication takes place is of great importance.

The context of communications

The context in which people communicate with each other influences the content and form of messages.

It is not usual for new acquaintances to converse about bladder and bowel function, but it is perfectly acceptable as an important discussion topic for a recently admitted patient and his doctor or nurse.

Someone doing an easy but monotonous job might receive commiserations, unless he was someone who had overcome great handicaps in order to achieve wage earning status, in which case he would be congratulated.

In a therapeutic community, an individual would discuss his problem at a group meeting to enable other members to help him overcome his difficulties, but a group discussion would be of little value to the person experiencing a cardiac arrest. In this instance, there is a need for minimal verbal interaction, and the swift and efficient implementation of a prearranged course of action.

A student nurse may well have ideas about changes in the care of a patient, but be unable to verbalise these adequately if she feels the ward sister would disapprove.

Learners could be presented with hypothetical situations and asked to suggest how communications might differ.

For example, a nurse has given food to a patient who was being prepared for anaesthesia, prior to electroplexy. How would Sister's communications differ when she was:

1. Speaking to the patient;
2. Speaking to the anaesthetist;
3. Speaking to the errant nurse.

A good clinical example is that of a report from the pathology department. The written document is concise and unaccompanied by other cues. The ward sister receives it, reads it, shows a good deal of change in her facial expression, and hands it to the doctor. He reads it, comments on its clinical significance, and goes to see the patient. The nurse and the doctor have composed their faces and explain to the patient that the results indicate that he will need a change in his treatment. Sister then explains to the junior student nurse, in simple terms, the significance of the laboratory findings. The written communication was sufficient for the experienced staff, the findings had to be translated into terms of treatment required for the patient, and the inexperienced nurse needed help to find significance in the written report.

Having been given an example suitable for her clinical area, the learner could then be asked to look for examples herself, and to note when written, oral and nonverbal components are involved.

When the learner is familiar with the aspects of communications outlined above and when she has gained a little clinical experience, she can begin to use her knowledge to increase communication opportunities with patients.

Communications in the clinical setting

The way in which knowledge of aspects of communications can be used will depend on the clinical area to which the learner is allocated.

An example is a ward for patients who have been resident in hospital for many years, and have grown old. There are many such patients in our psychiatric hospitals, and the long stay ward is their permanent home. The nurse learner will probably be involved in the care of a group of patients, and the clinical teacher can help her to employ her knowledge of communications while planning care.

Many elderly people have sight and hearing deficits, and it is wise to ensure that spectacles and hearing aids are provided where necessary. The nurse who uses her powers of observation can bring any such patient to the attention of the nurse in charge.

The nurse can look at patients' records to find out what shared experiences exist. Some patients have spent more time together than many members of families.

She can observe the social interactions taking place in the ward and ensure that her interventions will not impede any established activities which are beneficial.

Further information that she will find it useful to note includes patients:

1. With limited head and neck movement
2. With limited locomotor ability
3. Who are slow in speaking
4. Who tend to be solitary
5. Who tend to intrude on others
6. Who are over-active
7. Who are most at ease surrounded by space
8. Who are most at ease in close proximity to others.

She will also need to assess the ability of each of her assigned patients to be involved in social conversation with others.

Having assessed the communications difficulties, the learner will need to consider facilities and opportunities available for improving activities for the group.

High backed wing chairs are supportive and tend to reduce the impact of draughts, but they can act as barriers to conversations if those sitting in the chairs are unable to lean forward or turn their heads easily. The best use must be made of space and furniture, and this will probably involve the nurse in some furniture moving.

Someone who is unable to walk can be placed close to, and opposite another person with similar interests, but the chairs must be positioned so that they are pointing slightly away from each other. This enables pauses to take place, or even longer breaks, without difficulty, because in the resting position each individual will be looking away from the other, and yet only as small amount of neck or eye movement is needed to re-establish contact.

Care must be taken to ensure that personal space is not violated; it can be quite uncomfortable if chairs are touching and every slight movement made by one person is felt by the next. This is particularly important in those patients who have been observed to prefer solitude, or to need more space than most.

Arrangements must be made for those who have been together for many years, and enjoy each other's company, to continue to do so, and at the same time watch must be kept that no-one is overburdened by the company of someone who cannot be tolerated for long.

Some long stay patients find little to say once a conversation has been initiated, and this could be because of lack of recent stimulating experiences. It is possible for newspapers, television or radio to be used in constructive ways, to enable new topics of conversation to be broached, and the nurse can be encouraged to use her own imagination to increase interest. One way would be to take a general topic of interest, and plan to read from a paper, watch a television programme, and listen to a radio broadcast on that topic, with discussions in between. Topics such as the Royal Family, food and wildlife are some suggestions. A nurse who is interested in improving the quality of life of long stay patients would probably find such activities more useful and satisfying than merely switching on the television set and ensuring that everyone had a clear view.

The geographical situation of the ward could lend itself to increase in conversation. Flowers and trees can be lovely to look at and interesting to speak about. Patients might like to contribute stories about parks or the country from their childhood, or a once keen gardener might tell of his successes.

If the population of the ward is largely from the local area, local newspapers can be useful. Changes can be read about and commented upon, and reminiscences are usually not far behind.

People who are slow to respond may appreciate gentle prompting, or definite cues from the nurse. The teacher can help the learner in the initial stages by taking over some of the observations, for example, she could look for signs of fatigue or boredom, or distress in the patients, whilst the nurse is getting used to coping with communications which are tempered by paucity of information, and physical disabilities which interfere with eye gaze and facial expression, among other problems.

The nurse may need help in sustaining conversations once they have been initiated. Concentration spans tend to be shorter in old age, and social interaction is emotionally demanding for those who have grown unaccustomed to it.

It is easy for a nurse to become so accustomed to stimulating discussion that she overlooks the possibility of conversations being initiated by others. Even if a topic suggested by a patient does not have wide appeal, it is important to recognise the effect involved, and to take up the suggestion.

Of course, communications take place throughout the day, and many patients in long stay wards have no lack of verbal stimulus, but it is important to provide the best possible quality of life for all patients, and introducing more variety of conversation and a wider range of interests for short periods each day must be of value to those whose opportunities have been curtailed.

In addition to helping patients interact with each other, the nurse by this time will be more alert to the verbal and nonverbal communications of individual patients with whom she is working. It is not always possible, for example, for an elderly institutional-ised person to state clearly that she is not feeling well, but by being aware of the individual's usual behaviour patterns, unusual nonverbal cues as reduced eye gaze, increased isolation, and changed posture could indicate to the observant nurse that something untoward was happening to the patient.

The nurse's own communication abilities will be enhanced if she has the opportunity to present her nursing plan in written form. Practice, supervised by the ward teacher, will increase her skills, and this also applies to verbal reporting and other messages.

Awareness of the importance of observations, how to carry them out, and how to communicate the findings will enable the nurse to develop a sensitivity to changes in patients, and in others, and will enable her to provide suitable intervention.

Summary

1. Individuals learn how to communicate in various ways during the socialisation process.
2. Communications can be oral, written and nonverbal.
3. The context in which communications take place is important.
4. Human communications are complex, especially because of the variety possible in the use of language.
5. Humans are able to produce an infinite variety of messages.
6. Messages may be distorted or misunderstood because of the complexity of language and the fact that simultaneous verbal and nonverbal communications may be conveying different messages.
7. Language is used to exchange messages, but also to demarcate groups of people, and to exclude others.
8. Nonverbal signals can be used to support a verbal message, or to take its place, or to organise and mediate a social situation.
9. Nurse learners must be helped to understand features of normal communication by observations and experience in social situations.

10. Observation and participation in events in the clinical situation can increase understanding of the strengths and limitations of written, oral and nonverbal messages.
11. The learner needs experience in rephrasing messages under supervision, so that she becomes adept at changing words to those more appropriate for the situation, without distorting meaning.
12. It is important for the nurse to use professional terminology but to avoid the use of contractions and abbreviations which can be misunderstood.
13. Any clinical situation contains useful communication areas in which the nurse can gain experience.
14. An example of the use of communications knowledge and skills is given. Promotion of conversation among elderly long term residents in the aim.

Human relationship skills

There are several ways of conceptualising human relationships, but for the purpose of this chapter we can consider that, in the clinical situation, human relationships are social interactions aimed at achieving therapeutic benefits for patients.

This third group of skills relies heavily on the acquisition of observation and communications skills.

Whenever two or more people are together, some interaction takes place. Words are not a necessary component of this interaction, for as has already been noted a great deal can be communicated nonverbally. The more sophisticated the observation skills, the more cues can be noted. Thus, communication and observations are very important. Other important factors are:

1. The perception of status and roles of others involved in the interaction;
2. The individual's interpretation of the total situation, including changes which may occur during interaction;
3. The aims expected to be fulfilled by interaction.

It is useful to look at each of these three factors in turn, although it is important to realise that they do not function separately, and that they must be taken together with communications and observation skills.

The perception of status and roles

During the socialisation of the individual, he learns that society assigns various roles in accordance with the perceived status of the individual. Groups of people with a certain status are identified, for example, commuters, consumers, employers. Within the groups certain roles are expected to be fulfilled, for example, a commuter travels from his home to work in a different place. If he then changed to working near home, without travelling, he would no longer be a commuter, that is, he would have lost his status by not fulfilling his role. This, of course, is a very simple example, and each person in reality is cast in many roles which interrelate with each other. A woman may have the status of daughter, wife, mother, student, consumer, churchgoer, outpatient, among others. Certain kinds of behaviour are expected within each category, and she may have problems in attempting to fill all roles satisfactorily. Commitment to care of her husband and family may limit her role as daughter, and the behaviour involved in being a student could reduce time for her church activities.

The person coping with a number of roles successfully is given the additional status of being a good manager and this often leads to further roles being assigned. The person who manages well is admired, and perhaps envied.

The person who is unable to fulfil the roles assigned in socially satisfactory ways is not admired, and may be despised, rejected and thought to be inferior.

In some circumstances, only the status and roles important in particular situations are considered in assessing an individual. It may be that a man is greatly admired at work for his business acumen, but is unsuccessful in more intimate relationships with his family.

Over the years, the people who have cared for the mentally ill have been assigned different roles because of changing status. The attendants upon the insane acted in restricting capacities, aimed at containing socially unacceptable behaviour within the asylum. Gradually, attitudes to the sick and the helpers changed and psychiatric nursing is now respectable, although we have some way to go before suffering from a psychiatric illness becomes socially acceptable.

A patient's ability to interact with a nurse will depend to some extent on his perception of her status, and therefore, her role. His perception will be influenced by his preconceived ideas together with his assessment of the roles actually fulfilled in his current situation by the nurse. A nurse who is seen to take an active part in planning and delivering patient care will be perceived differently from one who fulfils a certain number of assigned tasks each day.

A doctor's ability to interact with a nurse will depend again on perception of roles. The doctor who sees himself as the sole authority on patient care, with the nurse carrying out his instructions, will bring different attitudes to interactions from the doctor who respects the nurse's authority in aspects of nursing care.

The nurse who has confidence in her own status, and her ability to fulfil the roles assigned, will bring to interactions with patients, doctors and others involved, different qualities from the nurse who sees her role as subservient to that of others.

It should be clear by now that the nurse's attitude to her job, and her competence in the clinical setting will influence interactions. It would seem obvious that relationships in the clinical situation are enhanced if the nurse is secure in an appreciation of her true status, and competent in the fulfilment of her roles.

The teacher can help the nurse to an understanding of status and roles by suggesting situations for observation and discussion. As in previous sections, it is thought useful to begin with common non-clinical situations, and the learner could begin by listing the role expectations she would have of various people she knows, for example, her mother, a shopkeeper, her father's employer, a young friend, a retired neighbour. As well as considering differences, it is important to consider similarities. The perception of roles of various people by different learners could be discussed, and this will reinforce the fact that people do show differences in perception.

Having looked at roles, it is then useful for the learner to consider how interaction with each person on her list differs, and try to find reasons for the differences. It is not implied that interactions are consciously made different, but what is being attempted is to make the learner more aware of the fact that differences do occur, and that there are reasons, some of which can be consciously identified and influenced.

Role play can be useful, with learners taking the part of people in different groups, e.g. a teenager talking to her parents, her friends, a prospective employer.

When the concepts of role and status in ordinary social settings are understood, the clinical situation will produce a number of different aspects to consider.

Patients, like other groups of people, tend to become categorised – the geriatrics, the long stay, the neurotics. Diagnosis requires that a name is assigned to a group of phenomena, and because the person is a patient to which a certain label is attached, particular-behaviours are looked for and expected. This concentration on the abnormal influences the way in which interactions develop.

If a learner can be encouraged to look at the normal areas of behaviour in addition to those highlighted by the diagnosis, she will learn to consider the whole person and her interactions will be influenced by a wider range of considerations.

An example would be a school teacher with an anxiety state. As well as the difficulties experienced because of the anxiety, she is still a person with an educated background, a consumer, a member of her church and family, and so on. The nurse will have a better understanding of the impact of the illness on the status and roles of this person than if she merely concentrated on the disorder itself.

From considering individuals who could be involved in inter-actions, the nurse can progress to considering the interactions themselves. This leads to the second factor mentioned earlier, the perception of the total situation.

The total situation, including changes occurring

The previous section concentrated on how individuals perceived others, but in human relationships the total situation involves the interactions which result from those perceptions.

If the expectations of all individuals involved in a social exchange are fulfilled, then the exchange will go smoothly. Approaches and responses will be made which lead without violent reappraisal into a further set of responses.

If, however, expectations are not fulfilled, then the normal social mechanisms do not apply.

For example, if a doctor's expectation is that a nurse waits for his instructions, then carries them out without further discussion, relationships will be smooth with the nurse who sees her role in those terms. The nurse who considers she has a contribution to make in determining the treatment programme, is unlikely to find interactions going smoothly with this doctor.

Human relationships therefore depend on more than individual perceptions of role and status. They also depend on the coincidence or otherwise of those views in all the people concerned.

A good source of unexpected behaviour for observation is television advertisements – they are used to provide impact because of their unexpectedness, but are useful for learning purposes to discover in what way the responses noted differ from those expected, and how the different behaviour influenced others in the situation. Advertisements are repeated and this is useful for checking observations.

A learner could be confronted with varied responses during role play, and asked to consider what she felt when faced with unexpected behaviour. At times the unusual is welcomed, and at times it could be irritating, annoying, or it could facilitate more important interactions.

All clinical situations provide opportunities for interaction with staff, patients and relatives.

It is worth noting which interactions make a nurse feel like producing more responses and which are inhibiting. In a ward meeting, a junior nurse may be contributing for the first time. If her contribution is received with signs to encourage her, such as smiles and nods, she will be inclined to speak freely whenever she has something to say. If, however, her contribution is ignored, or given less respect than those from other sources, she is unlikely to feel confident about further attempts. She is likely to have positive feelings towards those who encouraged her, and negative ones to those who did not.

If a nurse is given opportunity to assess her own behaviour, and discuss the implications with a teacher, she will be able to see how the influences of the total situation affect interactions. The perceptions of group members of each other, the purposes of the meeting, the pattern set by previous meetings, constraints such as time available, are all part of the total situation. If a ward meeting is held for the purpose of handing on information and instructions from the nurse in charge, the situation is different from that in which it is expected that information and suggestions are discussed.

Interactions are often less productive than they could be because the purposes are not clearly understood by all those concerned, or because the purposes are interpreted in different ways.

At the beginning of this section it was said that human relationships in the clinical area are interactions aimed at therapeutic benefit. If this is an acceptable way of viewing the interactions which take place, the nurse learner will be able to cope with problems such as poor responses or verbal aggression, because she will be able to view the event as part of the total therapeutic situation, rather than as a direct attack on herself.

It must be mentioned here than human relationships are not static, and the people involved respond to changes as well as to the original situation.

The total situation for the nurse learner based in a ward is a familiar one, and she has learned how to operate within that framework. For the patient, it is at first an alien environment, and he is unfamiliar with the behaviour expected of him. Add to this his anxieties about being ill, as well as the illness itself, and it is obvious that interactions are going to differ from those to which he is accustomed. The nurse is in a more confident and secure position, and this should be used for the patient's benefit.

If the nurse learner can be helped to understand the ways in which the total situation influences interaction, she will become more competent in human relationship skills, as she can apply this knowledge in her clinical encounters. It is essential that nurses of all ranks have opportunity in any clinical setting to discuss relationships within that situation. Discussion can clarify problems and lead to solutions. It can also confirm the nurse in her role, and help her to gain confidence in fulfilling it. The ward teacher would normally take part in such discussions, and would be of value in helping learners to a better understanding of factors influencing relationships.

Aims of interactions

It will be obvious from the most casual observations of human behaviour that variations occur due to the aims of social encounters.

It has been said earlier that the aim of clinical practice is to produce therapeutic benefit for patients. This seems rather one-sided, but if patients gain benefit then staff efforts are rewarded, so that benefit actually accrues all round.

The idea of 'therapeutic' value is very broad, and will have to be narrowed in accordance with the needs of each patient.

When nursing care is being planned, approaches to the patients, their problems and solutions, will be discussed. It is, of course, impossible to mention all possible approaches, but an example will be useful.

If a patient is found to have poor social skills, and one of the aims of care is to increase such skills, it is likely that specific situations will be used for this purpose. The morning greeting is an opportunity for an exchange of socially accepted phrases, together with eye gaze and smiles. This is a narrow focus on special aspects of a brief interchange – small in itself, but a step forward when success is achieved.

If the learner has clear ideas of what is expected from relationships within the therapeutic setting, she is better able to bring her knowledge and skills to produce most benefit.

The time worn exhortation to 'talk to the patients' shows good will but little else. Human relationship skills in ordinary social situations are developed over a lifetime of experience. Workers in the clinical area need an understanding of the components of the skills, practice in acquiring them and a knowledge of how they can be applied for the benefit of patients.

Nurses are involved in many encounters which do not include patients, e.g. with relatives or other workers; mutual benefit is expected from relationships and a clear idea of what to expect is helpful.

A staff discussion about a particular patient's care is not the time for a suggestion for improving the meals system. The same suggestion would be well received in a staff discussion of general amenities and provision for patients' welfare. The right contribution at the right time maintains expected role behaviour, reduces disruption which occurs following incorrect behaviour, and gives added prestige to the contributor. The discussion is moved further ahead, and progress is evident. This is the kind of interaction which is profitable for all. It comes from a competence in observation skills – to know when it is suitable to intervene; from competence in communications skills – to know how to make a contribution; and from competence in human relationships skills – to know what the aim of the interaction is and to make a contribution which will promote that aim with the given context of place and people.

Summary

1. Human relationships in the clinical setting can be conceptualised as social interactions aimed at achieving therapeutic benefits.
2. Human relationships are dependent on the acquisition of observation and communication skills.
3. Three additional important factors are identified:
   a. The perception of status and roles of others involved in interactions.

b. Interpretation of the total situation, including the influence of interventions.

c. The aims of interactions.

4. The behaviour expected of certain roles is mentioned, and reactions to expected and unexpected behaviours.

5. Suggestions are made for nurses to observe and examine social interactions.

6. Differences in perceptions of the role of the nurse are discussed.

7. The patient's ability to interact is discussed.

8. The importance of security in status is emphasised.

9. Suggestions are made for considering the behaviour of individuals in various circumstances.

10. The behaviour of people involved in social exchanges is discussed.

11. Ways of helping learners to examine interactions are explored.

12. The dynamic nature of interpersonal relationships is emphasised.

13. The influence of the total situation on interactions is discussed, particularly in relation to patients and nurse learners.

14. The aims of interactions are emphasised as being important to their progress.

15. Examples are given of good use of aims in interpersonal relationships.

SUGGESTED READING

Altschul, A. T. (1972) *Patient Nurse Interaction*. Edinburgh: Churchill Livingstone.

Argyle, M. (1967) *The Psychology of Interpersonal Behaviour*. Penguin Books.

Axline, V. (1971) *Dibs: In Search of Self*. Pelican Books.

Baron, R. A., Byrne, D. & Kantowitz, B. H. (1977) *Psychology: Understanding Behaviour*, Philadelphia: W.B. Saunders.

Berne, E. (1964) *Games People Play*. Penguin Books.

Pease, K. (1974) *Communication with and without words*. Vernon Scott Associates Ltd.

Powell, D. (1982) *Learning to Relate?* London: Royal College of Nursing.

Sprott, W. J. H. (1958) *Human Groups*. Pelican Books.

Stockwell, F. (1972) *The Unpopular Patient*. Royal College of Nursing.

Stuart, G. W., Sundeen, S. J. (1979) *Principles and Practice of Psychiatric Nursing*. St Louis: C.V. Mosby.

Towell, D. (1975) *Understanding Psychiatric Nursing*. Royal College of Nursing.

8

Fieldwork teaching

Fieldwork teaching techniques closely parallel those of clinical teaching. However, the fieldwork teacher continues to work as a health visitor with a caseload either in a geographically defined area or in attachment to a general practice. She normally has responsibility for one or two health visitor students during their course. The students attend the fieldwork teacher's place of work, and their studies are based on her workload. These differences in circumstances of fieldwork teaching compared to clinical teaching change the nature of the teacher–learner relationship. This chapter describes the special responsibilities of the fieldwork teacher and how the effective teaching of health visiting practice may be approached.

The development of fieldwork teaching

The need for a specially qualified health visitor to teach the practical aspects of health visitng was apparent from the inaugural meeting of the Council for the Education and Training of Health Visitors in 1962 (CETHV 1962–1983). Preparatory courses for fieldwork teachers initially lasted for two weeks. By 1982, courses consisted of six weeks of fulltime study spread over an academic year. On satisfactory completion of this first part of the course, the student proceeds to one year's supervised practice. The probationer fieldwork teacher is responsible during this time for one student health visitor. She is supervised throughout by a college health visitor tutor and a designated nursing officer or senior nurse. Each sends final reports to the College examination board at the end of the period. On receipt of satisfactory final reports, the fieldwork teacher is awarded the Certificate in Fieldwork Teaching. Thus, in addition to her health visiting certificate and other qualifications, the fieldwork teacher is highly qualified to teach health visitor students.

Admission requirements for the course

In addition to holding a health visitor's certificate, applicants must have at least two years' full-time (or equivalent part-time) experience in the United Kingdom as a practising health visitor. The full range of health visiting duties must have been undertaken normally in the year prior to the beginning of the course. Thus, specialist health visitors working solely with the elderly (for example) will not qualify for the course.

Selection is by written application to a training institution supported by a professional reference from the applicant's employing Health Authority, or Board (CETHV 1981). The fieldwork teacher training school also interviews the candidate. This provides the prospective fieldwork teacher with an opportunity to question and inform herself more fully of the nature of the course.

All courses were given initial approval by the CETHV (now UKCC) and follow common guidelines. Stronger emphasis, however, may be put on different topics by the various colleges.

The range of work

The fieldwork teacher may be based in an urban or rural area, working with a geographical caseload or attached to a general practice. Other duties such as running clinics and health education sessions are responsibilities she bears as part of her normal workload. She is physically separated from the main centre of teaching for her students, often by many miles. She is often isolated from other fieldwork teachers, and has only one or two student health visitors. To overcome this relative isolation, many fieldwork teachers link together to form tutorial groups. Alternatively, in some areas tutorial groups are formed with district nurse practical work teachers, G.P. trainers and others teaching students in the community.

The time specified for practical work by the UKCC is not more than one third of the academic part of the course. How this time is split up is decided by the college in discussion with the fieldwork teachers and in the light of past experience. This type of contact between college and the fieldwork teacher is regarded as important liaison by health visitor tutors. They are well aware of the difficulties involved in being responsible for a caseload and teaching a student simultaneously, so joint planning has great advantages. Besides liaison with the training school, the fieldwork teacher plans the student's programme and actively teaches the student the practical process of health visiting. Her evaluation of the student's progress (which takes place throughout the practical work) plays a part in the final assessment of the student's competence and suitability to qualify as a health visitor.

Areas of responsibility

Liaison with training school

Attending meetings at the college. Meetings for fieldwork teachers are held at regular intervals by the various colleges running health visitor courses. Normally, there is a briefing meeting at the beginning of the academic year for all the fieldwork teachers taking students. Here she can gather inforamtion about the previous year's students. The external examiner's special comments may be discussed, together with changes for the oncoming year. As a member of the academic team, the fieldwork teacher has a chance to put forward her own observations and ideas which can be discussed openly with her colleagues. She can also gain some insight into the philosophy of the particular course. Information received previous to this regarding her particular student may have been minimal, so this meeting may provide her with an opportunity to learn more about the student and her past professional experience before meeting her in the flesh. Fieldwork teachers may vary in the amount of background information on the student that they require. Some may argue that as a member of the teaching team the fieldwork teacher should have access to all the available information about her student. However, others argue that the information should be kept to a minimum, and name, age, previous experience and seconding or sponsoring authority is sufficient.

This latter policy, which is widely favoured, allows the fieldwork teacher to be more objective in her assessment of the student, and puts her less at risk of being influenced by the opinions and value judgements of others.

Initial meeting with students. The introductory meeting between the fieldwork teacher and her students normally takes place at the college. This meeting is important in settling the tone for the working relationship necessary for productive work during the year ahead. The fieldwork teacher uses her skills in establishing rapport with the students, and (in particular) listening to any problems which may arise. Transport difficulties often occur both in towns and the country, and special action may be necessary to resolve them.

The main aim of the meeting is to allow mutual introductions to take place. The fieldwork teacher should check whether the student knows how to find the health centre or clinic, and give directions as necessary. The meeting should be kept fairly brief yet an atmosphere should be created in which the student feels free to ask questions about areas that may be troubling her. This is vital to the development of the professional relationship.

Variations in interpretation and emphasis of syllabus

How it affects fieldwork teaching. Meetings at the college allow the fieldwork teacher to find out what academic work the students are expected to undertake, how different subjects are taught and assessed, and the place of various topics in the course timetable. This information enables the fieldwork teacher to plan a complementary practical teaching programme. Some colleges produce handouts in which they request specific practical experiences to be arranged each term; others will rely on verbal communications by the college tutors on visits to the practical work area, at the study days and business meetings held at college.

Meetings at the fieldwork teacher's base. It is valuable to all concerned if meetings of a largely tutorial nature can occasionally take place at the fieldwork teacher's base. It gives the college tutor an opportunity to get to know the fieldwork teacher individually and to understand the conditions under which she works; it aids the tutor giving tutorials in college to keep in touch with work at field level; and the tutor may have the chance to meet with nursing officers and other health visitors.

In order that maximum value is gained from the meeting, it is important to arrange a room where disturbances are unlikely. The aims of the meeting should be clarified with the tutor in the presence of the student. This ensures that all the participants have similar expectations. The student in particular will be reassured by this approach. She may be rather unsure of the purpose of the meetings and thus feel at a disadvantage, especially if she is to present a piece of work. After the tutorial the tutor will normally wish to see the fieldwork teacher and student individually. She will have already observed their interaction, and will have gained an impression of whether they are working together smoothly. The fieldwork teacher can discuss with the tutor means of approaching the teaching of practical work. She can also informally raise any queries she has regarding the progress of the student. Difficulties in relation to certain aspects of the syllabus, or in providing relevant practical experience for the student over the full range of health visiting, can also be discussed.

Occasionally, personality problems arise between the fieldwork teacher and student. Although they each have a responsibility to attempt to overcome them as far as possible, discussing the nature of the problem with the tutor may help in finding a solution. If the fieldwork teacher feels that she can no longer assess the student objectively or teach her sympathetically, then it is better that the student be given another chance with an alternative fieldwork teacher whenever possible. This occurs but rarely and should be sorted out early in the course, otherwise the student will have insufficient time to start new case studies. It is vital that the tutor with overall responsibility for the particular student is individually known to the fieldwork teacher, so that if problems occur regarding the student's progress, informal communications can easily be made.

Presentation of case studies with the student. The fieldwork teacher should be familiar with the contents of the CETHV publication *Guide-lines for Health Visiting Studies* (1983). The leaflet describes the objectives of the study visits to families, the number of studies required, their length, content and presentation format. Individual colleges tend to have their own interpretation of the guidelines, and the fieldwork teacher needs to be aware of any variations. This background information is best gained at first hand from the college tutor, as the student may well misinterpret what is expected. The thought of case studies often sends students into a panic, thus preventing them from listening properly! Group presentations of case studies with other fieldwork teachers, students and the tutor are very useful when they can be arranged. Several studies can be discussed and approaches to them compared and contrasted. The case studies are a very useful teaching tool together with the neighbourhood study, since the student has to crystallise her observations of the area and illustrate how she is attempting to work as a health visitor. The case studies and notes of families visited provide a focus for discussion between student and teacher. The aims of the visits can be planned in advance and the student given guidance.

The student's progress in practical health visiting can to a limited degree be monitored by the fieldwork teacher in her careful assessment of written work.

Linking service with education. Liaison with the training school at whatever level has important professional implications. Tutors are at risk of becoming enmeshed in an academic world with the emphasis on research, higher degrees and academic standards. This is an aspect of nursing which needs further development, as noted by the Committee on Nursing who said that 'Nursing should become a research-based profession' (HMSO 1974). Nevertheless the practical aspects of health visiting in promoting the health of the individual in the community should not be forgotten. The field-work teacher has a vital role here as a link between the health visiting service and the formal educators. She is in a position to question what is being taught in the college because she is able to analyse the practical experience available. She can inform the tutorial staff of difficulties which are occurring at field level, and how recent legislation is affecting the service in practical terms. This dialogue, valuable to both service and education, is dependent on good professional relationships which both sides should attempt to establish.

Group study days for fieldwork teachers. Study days facilitate good communications and relationships and are normally organised by the college. However, it may sometimes be appropriate to invite tutors to relevant in-service training courses to participate in discussions regarding educational and service problems.

Topics for college study days may be suggested by the fieldwork teachers, and new ideas are always welcomed. Subjects may include detailed discussion of recent government reports and the implications of recommendations for the health visiting service. Discussion and analysis of case and neighbourhood studies is useful, especially in the light of the external examiners' reports. The scope of study is enormously wide because health visiting is dynamic and changes to meet current health needs.

Study days can only go a short way towards updating fieldwork teachers. It is their own responsibility as professional workers to continue their education. Professional organisations and colleges run suitable courses which were often approved by the CETHV up to 1983 when this body was disbanded and its statutory functions assumed by the UKCC.

Planning the student's programme

Before the student's programme can be planned, certain information should be obtained. This should include the dates set by the college for the student's practical work, term dates and any college requirements for practical work planning.

Role of management. A meeting with the nursing officer concerned with training and other fieldwork teachers in the District is useful before planning a programme. This is particularly pertinent for new fieldwork teachers or for those new to a college. The nursing officer may have attended meetings at the college, and be able to assist in interpreting plans to meet the college requirements. She may wish to give an introductory session to the students explaining how the management structure operates from field level upwards. The nursing officer can discuss with the students her views of the health and social needs of the area covered by the Health Authority or Board. The health needs of such a large population will almost certainly vary from the relatively small population covered by an individual health visitor. Discussions of this nature with nurse managers are useful in helping the student place her neighbourhood and case studies into a wider perspective. Also, students gain first hand insight into how the lines of management operate and what the work of a manager entails.

The needs of the individual student. Prior information regarding the student's qualifications is necessary if successful forward planning is to take place. The student who has not worked in the community will need a longer introductory period than the student who has perhaps worked as a district nurse prior to starting the course. However, much information regarding the student's particular needs will only be highlighted after the fieldwork teacher and student have worked together and formed a professional relationship. This may take some while to be established, and exists when the student and fieldwork teacher are confident with each other and understand each other's role.

The former professional experience of the student is relevant to the speed with which she adapts to health visiting. The young student, straight from hospital nursing and keen to prevent ill health, may find promoting good health a very abstract concept. She may also have difficulty in settling into the apparently unstructured world of the community. Alternatively, the older student, perhaps with her own family now growing up, may feel quite confident in her relationship with mothers and young children. Although the advice this older student gives may be quite correct, her approach may be wrong as a potential health visitor. She may have difficulty in promoting individual choice and teaching the mother to select advice which enables her to meet her own health needs. It is only through observation of the practice of health visiting and discussion of the process with the fieldwork teacher that the particular learning needs of the student will be revealed.

Linking college work with practical work. The college will normally indicate to the fieldwork teacher either verbally or in writing which syllabus areas are being met each term. A logical progression of topics is followed. For instance, when teaching child development one starts with the newborn and progresses towards the schoolchild analysing each milestone en route. This close observation of young children early in the course will greatly clarify the different milestones in development and help the student remember them. In this way college teaching is facilitated by practical experience.

Special visits. Visits to local organisations which the student has discovered to be relevant to her neighbourhood study could be arranged by the student herself in many cases. She should keep the fieldwork teacher informed of the appointments she is planning to make. The fieldwork teacher's role is then to question the value of the visit in order to ensure the student has thought out her aims and objectives thoroughly. The over-enthusiastic student may arrange to visit too many of the organisations which proliferate in some twilight urban areas. This can be detrimental if overdone, detracting from time spent on the practical aspects of health visiting. The shy student may tend to avoid making her own approaches to organisations, and may thus need encouragement from the fieldwork teacher. Special visits need to be timed to coincide with college work and are appropriately arranged by the fieldwork teacher and college tutors when necessary.

Co-operation from colleagues. It is a very useful experience for students to spend some of their time with health visitors other than the fieldwork teacher. They can then observe how other professionals carry out the practice of health visiting. Although the broad principles of health visiting are shared, different personalities will approach similar tasks in different ways. Consideration of the work of psychologist and therapist Carl Rogers (1961) can give the student confidence in developing her own personal qualities within the framework of health visiting. Work with a variety of personnel prevents the student from forming a stereotyped view of health visiting. Other advantages include relieving the fieldwork teacher to enable her to concentrate on the second student if there is one, and allowing her to complete some of her outstanding work. When the fieldwork teacher is on holiday or attending a course whilst she has students assigned to her for practical work, she must give those collegues given temporary responsibility for the students detailed plans of what is expected of them. Although absences are unavoidable at times, it is unfortunate if the student misses teaching during her practical work. Experience which the fieldwork teacher is unable to offer from her own area of responsibility, such as school health and group health education, should where possible be provided by colleagues.

Linking with other fieldwork teachers is an alternative way of providing a range of practical work experiences. The CETHV Research Project on the Field Work Range of Experience (1975) showed that fieldwork teachers who linked together in groups to provide the full range of experience were successful.

Experience with other members of the primary health care team can also be included in the student's programme, so that she can observe and evaluate their special role.

Fieldwork blocks. When the student arrives at the fieldwork teacher's base at the start of a two or three week practical work block, it is reassuring for her to be presented with the objectives and a planned programme or timetable for the weeks ahead. This will enable the student to establish her location on specific days, and she can ascertain the time she has to make her own visiting arrangements. She may also wish to attend the local library in order to search out information. The timetable should be as flexible as possible, since if it is too rigid or crowded the student will have no room to manoeuvre and plan her own time. Responsible planning is an important part of health visiting practice, and the student will need tuition in this area.

Finally, when the student's programme has been planned one should check that the objectives of practical work are being fulfilled i.e. that the learning activities are focused on the practical experience of health visiting. This ensures that the student has a good basis on which to build when she eventually qualifies. Time should be set aside each day to discuss the student's daily work and observations. This is especially important after the student has been out visiting families on her own. Occasionally, a follow-up visit is necessary if the student has found health problems she was unable to solve. The responsibility of the fieldwork teacher to the family and the student should not be forgotten (Burr 1982).

Teaching the student

Fieldwork teaching is the active process of imparting information to a student in order that she may learn health visiting. Bloom *et al* showed in the *Taxonomy of Education Objectives* (1956) how learning was a sequential process in which past learning forms the basis for future learning. The fieldwork teacher needs then to plan her teaching on a hierarchical basis in order to bring about the required changes in her student's behaviour that learning requires. Instructional objectives as described by Mager in his work *Preparing Instructional Objectives* (1962) are a useful way of defining the behaviour that is expected of the student after teaching has taken place. Evaluation is based on the degree to which the student has achieved the specified objectives. Mager points out that if the student is given a copy of the instructional objectives the teacher may have little else to do! The student should be able to direct her own activities to these ends, and learning becomes relevant. This does not reduce the fieldwork teacher's role; she has to specify the objectives, which is not always an easy task, and be available as a resource, a critic, a demonstrator of skills and a counsellor.

Orientation of student to area and clinic or health centre

Introductions. The value of showing the student around the field-work teacher's base, introducing her to the other members of staff and giving her a place where she can leave her belongings safely and be reasonably comfortable when writing up her notes, cannot be stressed enough. Maslow, in his work *Motivation and Personality* (1954), put forward the idea of a hierarchy of basic needs which must be satisfied before self-actualisation can be reached. Maslow's work reinforces the reasoning behind orientating the student and making her feel welcome to the clinic before any teaching takes place and before she feels motivated to learn. Where possible, the student should be given her own desk or a point where she will not be in the way when she wishes to write up notes after her visits.

Observations and discussion of the neighbourhood. The neighbour-hood study continues as a vital part of practical work, since it forms part of the examinable material presented at the Part II qualifying examinations for health visitors. These examinations take place at the end of the supervised practise period, which normally occurs in an area other than the practical work area. Many students question the value of an extensive neighbourhood sudy in an area in which they are unlikely to be working as qualified health visitors. Hunt (1982) argues that the concept of neighbourhood is often artificial and value laden. Difficulties inevitably occur with statistics from official sources which overlap the fieldwork teacher's working area and do not coincide with it. Students are given very few families to study, so defining the neighbourhood in which they live would result in a small restricted study. The fieldwork teacher must aim to clarify the objectives of the study in order to aid the student in understanding its purpose. Tradionally, the neighbourhood study should demonstrate the student's understanding of aspects of sociology and social policy with regard to health and the social problems in the area. The student should be able to produce a neighbourhood study for any area in which she is working, and show how social facilities and housing stock can affect the lifestyles of families. It is important to help the student obtain up-to-date statistics particularly relating to health. Interpretation of information can be difficult, and so the student will need plenty of time to prepare and discuss her findings with the fieldwork teacher.

While the neighbourhood study remains in its present form as part of examinable material, the student will need aid when defining and planning relevant material. Alternatives to the neighbourhood study are under review. Some tutors suggest that students should be allowed to elaborate on the previous year's study. A special aspect of health visiting in an area could also be studied as a pilot research project. This latter idea might suit a graduate health visitor student with knowledge of social research and methodology.

When evaluating the neighbourhood study, the fieldwork teacher should consider how much value it has as a teaching tool and how relevant it is to learning health visiting practice.

Discussion of the student's observations. This is perhaps the most vital part of fieldwork teaching, as so much of the student's time is spent visiting families and individuals unaccompanied. Because of the nature of health visiting, the presence of a third person at an interview will alter the natural flow of conversation and rapport and so prevents accurate assessment. Generally therefore, such a presence is avoided and the student learns through evaluating her own performance. The fieldwork teacher needs to set aside time each day the student makes visits, in order to allow analysis of the visits to take place through joint discussion.

The student in the early stages will need to learn how to assess the needs of her clients. Through discussion, the fieldwork teacher can reinforce her teaching and guide the student towards making her own decisions regarding her aims for future visits. These would include consideration of the health needs of different groups of clients and how these needs can be met. The special expertise of the fieldwork teacher as a fully practising health visitor here comes into play. Her up-to-date and wide knowledge of the resources of the area reinforce her expertise. The aim of the fieldwork teacher is to question and interpret the student's observations, thus guiding her in the process of health visiting. This is a two-way dialogue with the student also asking questions and seeking explanations. The fieldwork teacher must learn to communicate clearly and help the student to build on her previous professional experience. Terminology used should be explained to the student, otherwise teaching will not be clearly understood. Jargon (which may be used liberally in health visiting) must be clarified, as failure to understand may hinder further learning. Tornyay, in her book *Strategies for Teaching Nursing* (1982), gives a good guide to questioning students in order to obtain the desired response. Fortunately, as a health visitor, the fieldwork teacher has a great deal of experience in the use of careful questioning.

Discussion with the student is the best way of finding out what knowledge the student possesses and gaining feedback on what has taken place during her visits. It is not sufficient merely to listen to the student's report or read her notes; questions, if skilfully formulated, can help students link theory with practice. Ideas can be explored, and the student and fieldwork teacher can work together towards a solution to problems. This in turn demonstrates clearly to the student her teacher's genuine interest in her and health visiting.

Selection of suitable material for teaching health visiting

Selection of families for study. When selecting families for the students to study, certain criteria should be used. The number of studies the student has to present at the Part II Examinations should be considered. The required number at the time of writing is two. The student needs to be able to observe the normal development of young children in some detail and in different types of families. Although families with problems may seem more interesting for a student, they may mislead her into thinking that health visiting is primarily concerned with crisis intervention. It is safer to select families who are reasonably well known to the fieldwork teacher. A family new to the area may have problems the student fails to recognise and this again may present unforeseen problems.

Problems encountered. Because of the geographical mobility of families in Great Britain, it is possible that one or two of those selected for the student's study will move during the academic year. Additional families should be allocated to allow for this. Sometimes families are not agreeable to being visited by a student despite her professional qualifications. When asked by the fieldwork teacher they may agree to the arrangement because of the good relationship they have with her, but later fail to make the student feel welcome. When this is apparent it is usually better if the student withdraws gracefully.

Briefing the families. Families and individuals react in different ways to the request that a student health visitor visit them over a limited period of time. There are a variety of ways of approaching this, and the manner adopted largely depends on the individual relationship between the families and the fieldwork teacher. Many fieldwork teachers prefer to meet the student prior to selecting and briefing the families so that some 'matching' can take place. It is important to stress to the families, however, that a student health visitor is already professionally qualified; the title 'student' can be easily misinterpreted particularly by elderly people.

Discussion with the student of relevant information before visits

Students need as much information and discussion as is relevant for them before meeting their assigned families. Unless the student has had previous experience of community work, she may be easily overwhelmed by certain aspects of home visiting such as poor housing conditions. Consequently, she is prevented from observing other health needs of a family unless briefed before the visit. Time spent out on practical work is brief, so it is important to maximise its value.

Introducing the student to families and individuals. Details of the student's nursing qualifications may help to enhance information about the education and training of health visitors. Many people are unaware that health visitors are nurses. There is no formal rule that the term 'student' has to be used, but it is important that the client is not misled.

Supervision of the student's record keeping. This is an important part of teaching health visiting practice. The student needs careful guidance regarding the maintenance of records. She has to learn how to write records succinctly, efficiently and conscientiously with due regard to maintaining confidentiality. The fieldwork teacher as a role model must ensure that her own records are in order. She should be able to demonstrate a workable system of recording her priorities and routine visits including the day-to-day management of a caseload. New developments in the technology of records and record keeping need also to be considered by the fieldwork teacher. A micro computer (suitably programmed) could give an immediate caseload profile. Hunt (November 1982) describes the usefulness of caseload profiles and analysis in giving a more representative picture of health visiting practice. Evidence could be provided of social needs in an area and visiting patterns reviewed. Much useful time is spent by health visitors in recording information in an antiquated way and thought should be given to how this time could better be used.

Provision of opportunities for observation. Observation of all aspects of health visiting should take place during practical work. The experience is relatively valueless unless the student is aware of the aims and objectives to be achieved. An afternoon spent in an immunisation clinic could be completely wasted unless the student is aware that she is expected to be able to answer certain questions afterwards. These might include describing where and under what conditions the vaccines are kept and relating the procedural questions asked before a vaccine is administered to the theory underlying the session. Discussion should take place afterwards with the fieldwork teacher, especially where local circumstances may differ from what has been taught in college.

The administration of the clinic or health centre. The student needs to understand how a clinic or health centre is organised in order to understand its complexity. The nursing officer and health centre administrator are the appropriate people to inform the student about this, and they should describe their roles. The student will need guidance in defining her objectives for this interview. The role of the clinic or health centre as part of the local neighbourhood should not be forgotten, and can be elaborated in the neighbourhood study.

Clinic sessions. The prospect of working as a health visitor in child health clinics can be worrying for students, since mothers there feel free to ask the health visitor many diverse questions. Students in this situation become aware of their need to learn the practical aspects of infant feeding. Confidence can be established by allowing them to sit with the fieldwork teacher and other health visitors and participate where possible in the interview. Teaching difficulties can occur in clinic sessions as the latter are often busy times, and there is little opportunity for follow-up discussions. Mothers may wish to discuss personal matters which the presence of the student can inhibit. It is advisable that the student makes a note of advice she does not understand, and this can be discussed later. She should also be alert to times when she should withdraw from an interview.

Eventually the student will be able to interview mothers on her own during child health clinics. The fieldwork teacher should be in the vicinity and available to be called on for advice. It is important to give this responsibility to the student when she is ready for it, normally in the second or third term depending on previous professional experience. The student by then has a pool of knowledge to call upon in answering the many queries which can arise. In other clinics, such as those run for ante-natal mothers, the special role of the health visitor needs to be demonstrated. The student who is a registered midwife can easily regress into her former role in a familiar situation and forget to be aware of the health visiting aspects.

Screening tests. Practice in performing hearing tests, tests for vision and other developmental screening procedures may only be possible during student practical work. The student needs to be given the opportunity to become proficient in the methods used. The fieldwork teacher should demonstrate the various tests, and so must ensure she is proficient and up to date herself in the latest techniques. Observation of a proficient medical officer or general practitioner may also be useful.

Practical techniques. With the advent of prepacked milk feeds and separate milk kitchens in maternity and paediatric departments, many health visitor students will have had only minimal experience of making up infant feeds. It is therefore time well spent if the student can practise making up feeds under supervision. She should compare the instructions for mixing different types of milk powder and compare costs of the feeds available between the chemist and the clinic.

In addition, students who have gained only an obstetric certificate may need to be given extra tuition regarding advice and techniques for mothers who are breast feeding. Contact with groups such as the National Childbirth Trust and La Lêche may also be useful.

Putting a napkin on a baby, practical details of napkin hygiene and skin care are a few procedures of which the student may feel unsure, and she may appreciate some practical experience. This will involve either finding a willing mother and baby or spending a short time in a day nursery. It may seem surprising that potential health visitors are lacking in these basic skills, but practical work can fill the gaps.

Referral. During the planning stage the fieldwork teacher may arrange for the student to visit professional colleagues in other sections and departments such as the local area team of social workers. These contacts are valuable in the early part of the course to aid the student's understanding of their different roles in the community. Later, as the student's case studies are under way, and she is involved professionally with the families, referral to other agencies may need to take place.

In the early stages telephone contact is frequently made, and this is good experience for the student since some of the less experienced students may exhibit a degree of nervousness when first using the telephone professionally. Speaking on the telephone to unknown people about clients of whom one has only limited knowledge can provoke anxiety, particularly if privacy is lacking. The fieldwork teacher should remember this if the student appears reluctant to make telephone calls, and she should help her to plan logical telephone conversations with the relevant agency or nursing officers. Aspects of confidentiality need emphasis here, as it is easier inadvertently to break confidence in a telephone conversation than in a report or letter. Telephone contacts are frequently made by health visitors and assume an important part of the role, so it is necessary that the student becomes proficient in this. Selecting the correct agency for referral involves a considerable knowledge of the services available and the role boundaries of the health visitor and other personnel. The ability of the student to produce a correct referral plan for a family or individual shows that she has been able to synthesise and evaluate the information she has obtained.

Attendance at case conferences. Where possible it is useful for the student to attend at least one case conference during practical work, particularly if it concerns a family with whom she is familiar. Case conferences vary in their purpose and degree of formality. Since they now form an ever increasing part of the health visitor's workload, the student should feel confident of the role of the health visitor in relation to various families and individuals. She should be able to express this both in writing and verbally at a case conference, and be able to discuss her role with the client. The role of the nursing officer in providing support and advice to the health visitor is most important.

Provision and observation of health education sessions

Teaching the individual. Provision of opportunities to observe individual health teaching takes place throughout health visits and clinic sessions. The subtlety of the teaching may escape the student's notice in the early days of practical work, and techniques for this should be brought to her attention. She should be able to recognise how teaching takes place through discussion with the mother or individual, building on the client's existing knowledge and enabling her to interpret her previous experience. The 'art' of health visiting is evident during home visits; that is, the interplay of skills and knowledge that the health visitor possesses which enable her to promote health.

Teaching groups. The prospect of group teaching can be met with enthusiasm or sheer dismay by students. Their attitude depends on their past experience, their personalities and their individual interest. It is quite normal to feel some anxiety before a teaching session, so reassurance is helpful. Observation of various types of health education sessions should take place before active participation, and this forms an important part of the range of fieldwork experience (CETHV 1975).

When observation and teaching experience cannot be provided at the fieldwork teacher's centre, linking with other centres or fieldwork teachers should be considered. Where there is impossible the college may be able to make alternative arrangements.

It is preferable for the student to have met the group she is to teach and to have participated in discussion with them sometime before the session takes place. The teaching topic must be within the student's abilities and this depends on her stage in the course. It is usually desirable that the teaching practice is given in the second term when the student should feel fairly confident talking about the health visitor's role. The student will need adequate notice of the teaching topic in order to prepare her notes and obtain any visual aids necessary. This may also be the right time to arrange a visit to the Local Health Education Department. The visit then has a firm objective, as the department may be able to help the student in her preparations for teaching. However, the general aim for the student of discovering the functions of the department should not be forgotten. Guidance on planning material and selecting a suitable teaching method should have been given in college. The fieldwork teacher should be aware of the student's objectives for the session before supervision and assessment takes place.

Assessment of group teaching. In assessing the preparation of material, the fieldwork teacher should check that it is up to date; that it covers the topic; and that it is organised in a logical sequence. The room available should be made comfortable and free from trailing flexes if a projector or any other electrical equipment is to be used. The student's rapport with the group should be evaluated, as should her ability to cope with their responses and questions. The student's overall teaching ability is often difficult to assess, as much depends on her previous experience. It is important for the student and fieldwork teacher to spend some time evaluating the session together afterwards. This gives the student an opportunity to explore her own teaching ability and to pinpoint areas where improvement is needed. Runswick and Davis, in their book *Health Education Practical Teaching Techniques* (1976) provide a straightforward guide to planning teaching for health education purposes. This is useful to both the student in her preparation and delivery and to the fieldwork teacher in her assessment.

School Health Service experience. The full range of responsibility of the heath visitor in the school health service varies according to the policy of the Health District and the individual school. Since the health visitor student is being trained to work anywhere in the United Kingdom, she must be aware of all the responsibilities of school nursing.

School work is frequently delegated to school nurses who work directly with a designated nursing officer. This may mean that observation of and participation in medicals, cleanliness inspections and possibly some educational sessions, take place under the supervision of school nurses. Despite this, the student health visitor will need to know how sessions are organised and what they set out to achieve. Since the range of direct health visitor involvement in the school health service is so diverse, the student should also be able to discuss the evaluation of the service in its present form.

The student should be able to demonstrate that she is able to link her observations with government reports such as *The Report of the Committee on Child Health Services*, (1976). This will involve analysis of the recommendations made and comparison with practical aspects of both the health visitor's work and that of the school health service.

Health visiting skills. Teaching the interpersonal skills of health visiting is perhaps the most difficult part of fieldwork teaching, since in practice it is not possible to isolate one skill from another. For the student, however, the skills are demonstrated by the role model of the fieldwork teacher during practice, and through analytical discussions before and after interviews with clients. Observation of the student when interviewing will almost certainly alter her spontaneity in relation to the individual client. It is doubtful whether attempts to assess interpersonal skills in this way are of value. However, feedback from the student and even from the client can help towards assessment in this difficult area.

Bloom (1964) gives a basis for setting objectives in order to assess affective changes in the individual.

Achieving changes in attitudes and values takes more time than that available to the student in practical work, so assessment in this area needs to be approached with reservation. However, the student should be able to demonstrate that she is developing the necessary interpersonal and observation skills used in health visiting, and that she accepts the values implied.

Teaching the skills in organisation and planning. Practical health visiting skills such as record keeping and report writing need practice, constructive criticism and guided discussion from the fieldwork teacher. Similarly, the organisation and management of a caseload should be demonstrated and linked to the setting of priorities. The fieldwork teacher needs to be able to demonstrate knowledge of the vital statistics and other information concerning the area where she is working, and show the student how this knowledge is an essential part of health visiting practice.

One way of helping the student learn how to manage a caseload is to give her some responsibility for a small number of families over and above those selected for her case studies; between 10 and 20 families is quite sufficient. The student can then devise an index system or 'birth book' for her mini-caseload, and decide the order in which they should be visited. The fieldwork teacher should guide the student in this and retain overall responsibility for the families, in particular during the student's absence. The advantage of this system is that the student has the opportunity to observe the dynamics of caseload at close quarters. The disadvantages are that the fieldwork teacher may not have suitable families to hand over to the student, and indeed it may not be appropriate for all students to undertake this responsibility. However, during the third term most students feel ready to do some routine visiting in order to consolidate what they have learnt.

Evaluation of the student's progress.

Report writing and assessment. Assessment of the student by the fieldwork teacher takes place continually throughout practical work. The nature of health visiting does not lend itself to a structured timed assessment, as in general nurse training, so reports of the student's progress are necessary. Normally, guidelines for reports are issued by the college at the various points when they are required during the academic year.

These reports play a vital role in deciding whether a student finally qualifies as a health visistor. They can well alter the balance in either direction in the case of a borderline candidate. The completion of report forms is not then just a ritual. When completed, they are carefully read by the college tutors and retained for presentation at the final meeting of the examiners.

In writing the final report, the guidelines of the particular college should be followed but additional topics may also need thought by the fieldwork teaacher. Forms can be restricting when assessing an individual in that they can constrain the range of evaluation. The Nuffield Foundation *Report by the Group for Research and Innovation in Higher Education* (March 1972) suggests in section III(v) four target areas for evaluation:

1. Knowledge and problem solving ability
2. Personal characteristics
3. Skills
4. Self education abilities

Knowledge and problem solving ability should be increased as the academic year progresses, and it is the application of knowledge that is crucial in assessment. Acceptable personal characteristics are very important for a health visitor, and are considered carefully when applicants are initially interviewed. However, interviews are not a foolproof means of selection, so the fieldwork teacher has an important role in assessing whether a student is suitable. The ability to build up professional relationships and to understand their scope and limitations is sought. Desirable personal qualities include reliability, confidence, ability to use initiative and sensitivity towards both clients and colleagues. The skills used in health visiting include observation, assessment, organisation and planning, evaluation of work and the ability to communicate and teach group health education. The assessment of the student's self-education ability indicates how the student may develop when qualified. Does the student continue to study and use the library when out on practical work blocks? There are difficulties inherent in making assessments of a non-procedural nature. The fieldwork teacher must first establish the criteria for an acceptable level of performance and then compare it with her own student's performance. One must be as objective as possible. It is now usual for the student to see and comment upon her report before it is sent to the college, and because of this there may be a tendency to be more lenient. With the so called 'average' student this is relatively unimportant. However, in the case of students who do not appear to be suitable as health visitors, reports must be written accurately in order to protect professional standards. The fieldwork teacher should strive to become aware of her own idiosyncracies. External forces may also affect her judgment, such as expectations of the college tutor who will read the report. The halo effect can occur and prevent objective assessment, and thus a generally good or generally poor impression of a student can influence the teacher's view of specific aspects of the student's work.

Similarly, logical errors can occur; if the student is good or poor in one area, she may seem to be good or poor in other aspects. The sex of the assessor and student can also exert influence. The feminine gender has been used throughout this chapter, but men are entering health visiting, although few in number. The male health visitor student is vulnerable to incorrect assessment, because he is in a minority group and expectations of his progress may be altered.

Completion of report forms requires concentrated thought, and sufficient time should be allowed for this. They are unable to provide an absolute standard, but they can draw the attention of the student, the fieldwork teacher and the college tutors to areas of weakness and strength.

Counselling and support. During the academic year the fieldwork teacher and student work very closely together; this normally leads to the establishment of a good rapport between them. It is inevitable that sometimes the student may feel under pressure resulting from the quantity of new material to be learned and the prospect of examinations. The fieldwork teacher is in an ideal position to give the student the individual support she needs in order to encourage her in her work. Where problems arise of an academic or personal nature, the fieldwork teacher may well find herself in the position of a counsellor which will draw upon many of the skills used in health visiting. However, as Sheahan (1976) notes in his paper on 'Continuous assessment, guiding and supporting', the student may hesitate to be frank with a teacher who has to write a report about her in case this prejudices her future.

Professional development

The continuous process of education. The nature of fieldwork teaching demands that the health visitor keeps up to date with new information and professional developments in health visiting and allied fields. This is a responsibility the fieldwork teacher holds not only to herself and the public, but also to her colleagues and the next generation of health visitors whom she is helping to train and educate.

Facilities available for study leave and payment of expenses for those wishing to attend post-registration study courses and conferences are not always made known to staff in the National Health Service. It is up to the fieldwork teacher to assess and articulate her own needs to nursing management and to bodies who provide courses. Awareness of changing needs can be acquired through reading the nursing press and professional journals and attending study days where professional discussion takes place. Taylor (1975) in her paper 'Continuing Education for Nurses' lists six main objectives that the nurse should be set, in order that she should:

1. Remain competent
2. Develop as an individual
3. Keep abreast of new developments
4. Learn new skills and techniques
5. Implement research findings
6. Prepare for work in special areas and for leadership in general.

The general objective is that she should maintain and improve the quality of patient care.

Health visiting practice covers many different aspects of health, so it is impossible for an individual to read all the literature published. The dilemma posed by the volume of information is partially solved by reading nursing, medical and health visiting journals. In this way the reader benefits by having information preselected as professionally relevant brought to her attention.

To develop as a fieldwork teacher evaluation of one's teaching is essential. Fundamentals should be considered regularly, such as whether one's aims and objectives are achievable and realistic and whether modifications to planning and teaching are necessary. There are no absolute criteria for methods of evaluation, but in most circumstances the most severe and knowledgeable critic will be oneself. Students and the college tutors can provide but limited feedback. It is a teacher with a mind that is alert to new ideas and who is willing to try them who is the most successful.

REFERENCES

Bloom, B. S. (Ed.) (1956) *Taxonomy of Educational Objectives. The Classification of Educational Goals. Handbook 1: Cognitive Domain.* (New York: David McKay Company Inc.) Harlow: Longman.

Bloom, B. S., Krathwohl, D. R. & Masia, B. B. (1964) *Taxonomy of Educational Objectives. The Classification of Educational Goals. Handbook II: Affective Domain.* Harlow: Longman

Burr, M. (1982) *The Law and Health Visitors.* London: Edsall.

Council for the Education and Training of Health Visitors (1983) *Guidelines for Health Visiting Studies.* Curwen Press.

Council for the Education and Training of Health Visitors (H. M. Williams) (1975) *A Report of the findings of a small investigation carried out on fieldwork range of experience.* London: CETHV Publication.

Council for the Education and Training of Health Visitors (March 1981) *The Fieldwork Teacher Courses.* London: CETHV Publication.

Department of Health and Social Security (1972) *Report of the Committee on Nursing* (Chairman: Professor Asa Briggs). Cmnd 5115, Section 370, p. 108. London: HMSO

de Tornyay, R. (1982) *Strategies for Teaching Nursing,* 2nd edn. New York: Wiley.

Hunt, M. (1982a) A critique of the neighbourhood study in health visitor training. *Health Visitor,* 55, 10, 521–525.

Hunt, M. (1982b) Caseload profiles – an alternative to the neighbourhood study. *Health Visitor,* 55, 11, 606–607.

Mager, R. F. (1962) *Preparing Instructional Objectives.* Belmont, California: Lear Siegler, Inc./Fearon Publishers.

Maslow, A. H., (1954) *Motivation and Personality,* Ch. 5. New York: Harper & Row

A Report by the Group for Research and Innovation in Higher Education (1972). *A Question of Degree,* assorted papers on assessment Section III(v). *Evaluation of Student Progress:* M. D. Program, Faculty for Medicine, McMaster University, Canada: The Nuffield Foundation.

The Report of the Committee on Child Health Services (Chairman: Professor S. D. M. Court) (1976) *Fit for the Future.* Cmnd 6684. London: H.M.S.O.

Rogers, C. R. (1961) *On Becoming a Person.* Boston: Houghton Mifflin.

Runswick, H. & Davis, C. (1976) *Health Education Practical Teaching Techniques.* Aylesbury, Buckinghamshire: HM & M Publishers.

Sheahan, J. (1976) Education-9, Continuous assessment, guiding and supporting. *Nursing Times*, 72, 1650.

Taylor, C. R. (1975) Continuing education for nurses. *Nursing Times* (Occasional Paper), 71, 29.

FURTHER READING

Anderson, D. C. (1979) Health Education in Practice. Croom Helm.

CETHV (1982) Principles in practice. London: CETHV

Eweles, L. & Shipster, P. (1981) One to One. East Sussex A.H.A.

Pettes, D. (1972) Supervision in Social Work. N.S.W.

Robinson, J. (1982) An evaluation of health visiting. London: CETHV.

9

Paediatric clinical teaching

Paediatric clinical teaching offers a wide range of opportunities in a specialist field. It involves the education of nurses, children and their parents, under circumstances that may be strange to all of them.

The teaching of paediatric care in hospitals takes place mainly in two distinct areas – the general hospital with a relatively small paediatric unit, and the specialist children's hospital. The clinical teacher must be able to adapt teaching methods to suit not only these different areas in paediatric nursing, but also to suit the varying requirements of different types of students. These students generally fall into two main categories: those who have an eight week allocation to fulfil the requirements for their final examination, i.e. the students studying for Enrolment, General Registration, and degree courses; and those students studying paediatrics for a longer period, i.e. for integrated general Registration and registration for Sick Children's Nursing and the post-graduate courses for Enrolled and Registered general students. Both long and short stay students may be found in each type of hospital.

Nurses starting their eight week allocation will probably do so with a minimum of paediatric knowledge, regardless of the stage that they have reached in their course. These learners require a general knowledge of paediatrics. The introductory week in a modular system of training should provide for the learner the opportunity to observe children in a more natural environment, for example, play groups, nursery schools, 'well baby' clinics, toy libraries or any other facility the clinical teacher can organise with community staff. This will give the learner more confidence in approaching this new and different type of nursing. When she comes to work on the ward, the nurse will need considerable help in learning to give basic nursing care to the sick child. This means that the amount of supervision and teaching required from the clinical teacher and trained ward staff is great. While she progresses through the module, new procedures needing further explanation and support frequently arise.

The more senior among the learners must be told to expect as much supervision as the juniors; paediatric nursing is to different that until shown the correct methods and skills they may be unable to carry out even simple aspects of care. Experience gained over previous years in different clinical areas is not necessarily applicable. Even recording an infant's temperature bears little resemblance to the adult procedure; and once this is mastered, replacing the napkin requires the combined arts of origami and gentle persuasion!

Unless nurses are made aware that they will be fully supervised while so many new techniques are learned, they may suffer a loss of self-confidence and possibly feel resentment towards others more junior who have a greater knowledge since they are near the end of their allocation. These problems may be aggravated for those nurses nearing final examinations who have built up their knowledge and confidence on the general wards over the previous years, only to be faced with something completely new when entering the paediatric unit. In such cases, support and encouragement must be given.

During the introductory week, to help overcome the newness of the subject, it will be helpful for the clinical teacher to introduce the learners to the ward, giving them a chance to familiarise themselves with the general layout. Handouts showing ward routine and objectives of their period of allocation should be given (for the latter, see Figure 9.1). Demonstrations of basic procedures, for example admission of a child to the ward, will again help to increase the nurse's confidence and ability in carrying out her work as a children's nurse.

The approach to teaching nurses on the four-year integrated course, leading to general Registration and Sick Children's Nursing, will be slightly different. Usually these nurses would be attached to a children's hospital for their paediatric training and to a general hospital for adult nursing. Often these hospitals are in the same group. The nurses will again require a lot of supervision at first, but since they are not only new to paediatrics but also to nursing in general, all procedures will be totally strange. Therefore a greater amount of teaching of both practical skills and theoretical knowledge is required in the introductory period.

A nurse who has done some general nursing has had time to learn to cope mentally with being close to illness and death. Even

On completion of your practical nursing experience in this area area you should be able to:	Initial

1. Have spent 5 days in the community observing children in their normal environment and have completed the appropriate check list of experience.
2. Receive and admit children recording the necessary particulars and relevant nursing observations.
    Talk to and advise parents.
    Know and be able to arrange the appropriate resources for continuing after care.
3. Take and record rectal temperatures.
4. Collect specimens for laboratory investigations including:
    urine
    nose swabs
    throat swabs
    and state reason for these.
5. Change babies' nappies.
6. Bath babies
7. Demonstrate your knowledge of infant feeding by:
    a. observing and feeding infants by bottle or tube,
    b. discussing the principles of breast feeding,
    c. sterilizing feeding equipment and discuss the principles involved in this,
    d. calculating the energy requirements.
8. Administer drugs to children
9. Demonstrate your understanding of the care given to children receiving intravenous infusions and blood transfusions by
    a. stating the reasons for the infusion/transfusion,
    b. relating the safety involved,
    c. ensuring the correct rate of flow,
    d. checking and changing the pack of fluid,
    e. recording accurately the amount received,
    f. making knowledgeable and accurate nursing observations during the infusion/transfusion and stating the reason for these,
    g. describing the causes of major and minor reactions.
10. Demonstrate, either in practice or by verbal or written description, your understanding of the specific nursing care given to children who undergo:
    tonsillectomy
    or who are suffering from:
    thalassaemia
    gastro-enteritis
    pyloric stenosis
    burns/scalds.
11. Give the specific preparation and after care for children who have cardiac catheterisation. Observe this procedure being performed.
12. Give the appropriate physical and psychological nursing care for children who are terminally ill: including care of their parents.
13. Assemble the necessary equipment and perform last offices.
14. Attend a discussion group with the child psychiatrist.
15. Observe the work of the school teachers and play therapist and discuss their roles in hospital.

Fig. 9.1 Ward learning objectives for a particular paediatric ward

so, coming to a children's ward can still cause considerable distress. For a newcomer to nursing, entering a specialist children's hospital (which is likely to receive the most severely ill children), the effect can be completely demoralising. The clinical teacher must be able to discern such problems and give sufficient support until the nurse is able to deal with her own emotions. In many hospitals, it may be possible to provide a support team of a social worker and child psychiatrist to help the nurse to cope with the problems and needs both of the child and its family, and herself.

It should be noted that in recent examinations, emphasis is put on the psychological care of the child in hospital. A clinical teacher should be able to assist the nurse in learning how to give this supportive care by ensuring that while she is demonstrating practical procedures, a full awareness is shown, in her conversation and attitude, of the child's psychological needs.

While the learners progress, the role of the clinical teacher changes. As a knowledge of the subject is gained the emphasis changes from acquiring practical skills to the application of theory to practice. Causes and effects of disease and the resultant problems, child psychology and physiology, which are only touched on as necessary during the first few weeks, can now be dealt with far more fully. For a nurse working in a hospital where children with rarer conditions are nursed, or working in, say, a neonatal or intensive care unit, the knowledge gained will be beyond the scope of any immediate examinations, but will nevertheless be invaluable in her later career. In addition, the clinical teacher needs to teach the subject in depth in order to stimulate and maintain the nurse's interest throughout a lengthy course. Sight, however, must not be lost of the requirements of the examination, and time must be allowed for consolidation and revision at regular intervals. More advanced students may be given a topic (for example – care of the child with cystic fibrosis, asthma, or gastro-enteritis), on which to give a ward tutorial under the supervision of the clinical teacher. One of the best ways of learning a subject is, after all, to teach it.

Post registration students – both Enrolled nurses and Registered nurses starting a six or thirteen month specialist course – already possess a grounding in paediatrics from their previous training. Having enjoyed working with children, they have chosen further to develop their skills in this field. Often, though, they have worked as staff nurses, sometimes even on children's wards, and have confidence in their abilities through qualifying and holding a position of responsibility. Hence the thought of going back to school may prove an obstacle, and the clinical teacher may find there is slight resentment on the students' part at being taught again. Because different hospitals use different techniques for basic skills (the writer has been taught nine ways to bath a baby – with each the baby comes out clean!) the students must be retaught so that they may conform to the individual hospital's mores.

It should be explained suitably to them that, although no one is decrying what they have been taught in the past, they will in due course be teaching more junior learners; it is therefore unfair to confuse these learners with different methods. Then it is more likely that they will be prepared to accept their role as students without ill-feeling.

It may also be difficult for post registration students to accept that their responsibility for ward administration is reduced, particularly when the person in charge of the ward may have no more experience than themselves. The student may feel herself to be in an awkward position, but the clinical teacher can alleviate the problem by maintaining the student's self-confidence and utilising her knowledge and experience in the teaching programme for the less advanced learners. The introduction of total patient care is of benefit to children, parents, and nursing staff. With this scheme for the provision of care, students assess, plan, deliver and evaluate the nursing care which they each give under supervision to a small number of children. It therefore develops in the learners both a sense of achievement and a sense of responsibility.

Having considered the different types of student with whom the clinical teacher will have to cope we can now consider paediatric teaching generally. When one is teaching totally new skills, for example infant bathing and feeding, to learners who are not confident in handling children, it is best for the teacher to *demonstrate* first, discussing the technique at the same time, while the learner observes and asks any pertinent questions. The learner, who will gain simply by watching the handling of an infant by an experienced person who acts as a role model, should then perform the same skill for another infant while the teacher observes. The sooner the learner does this after the initial demonstration, the less likely it is that the teacher will have to stop the learner to correct her. When someone is carrying out a technique for the first time, it is inevitable that she will have to concentrate on the job in hand, and she will therefore tend to stop if discussing points or asking questions. The longer the period between the demonstration and trying out the technique, the more questions are likely to arise, and therefore the longer the job is drawn out – leaving, for example, a damp infant suspended in mid-air while the learner asks 'Is this the best way to handle him?'

It is inevitable that on occasions a learner will have to be taught in front of parents, since they are frequently resident in paediatric units. This has to be done with great care to ensure that the learner's self-esteem is not lost, and that the parents' confidence in the nursing staff is maintained.

To do this, the clinical teacher should be aware of the knowledge the learner has already acquired, and should question her on it (a good technique at any time to increase self-confidence). She can then introduce new information into the conversation for the learner to assimilate.

These new ideas can be reinforced by asking questions at a later date. New information can also be put across in the form of leading questions, making it appear that the learner already knows the facts: for example, she may be asked, 'A thermometer with a blue bulb is used for taking rectal temperatures, isn't it?' . . . . to which the learner will answer . . . 'Yes'.

This should not normally present any problems, as long as the nurse realises she must be very clear in her own mind about what is required before trying to explain it to someone else. Occasionally, parents will be encountered who are reluctant to be taught, if not actually resentful. Where simple tact and persuasion fail, one course still open is to educate them without their realising it. The clinical teacher can teach a nurse the necessary points while in the presence of the parents.

In the more specialised paediatric hospitals, it may be rare to find children suffering from relatively uncomplicated medical conditions such as asthma, appendicitis, fractures, adeno-tonsillectomy, non-accidental injuries and the like, a knowledge of which is required for final examinations. While book learning is no substitute for practical experience, unfortunately it is, in such cases, the only answer. Ward tutorials on such subjects should be arranged, and in such a way that as many learners may attend as often as is possible. From the writer's past experience, it has been found that attendance is good since there is concern on the students' part about being able to cover the full syllabus. Report time can then be used correctly for discussing the care of children currently in the ward.

Whereas most nurses before commencing training have a pretty fair idea of what constitutes a normal healthy adult, not many have the same preconception concerning children. An insight into this may be gained by attending the local playgroup, nurseries, or schools. The leaders of such groups are usually extremely helpful. The clinical teacher can then point out how children play and interact at different ages and how their physical and mental abilities develop. To help a learner recognise the milestones in a child's development in relation to age, it is a good idea to encourage the learner to speak to and observe a child at play and to try to guess its age. The child itself will probably enjoy the game! A questionnaire as in Fig. 9.2 (which applies to the 2 to 8 age group) is also a useful basis for debate after observing a group at play. The students should write comments on as many of the questions as they find relevant to the age group they are visiting. Then, if different students have visited different groups, a general picture can be built up of milestones in development during the subsequent discussion. Many children's departments nowadays employ a full-time play therapist. Her help can be invaluable to the student in learning to assess progress or regression of children in her care.

---

1. Are any children still in nappies?
2. Can the children carry on a conversation with you?
3. How far have they progressed in sentence construction?
4. What types of games are the children playing?
5. At what age do they start playing in groups?
6. For how long can they concentrate on one game?
7. How do they hold a small object?
8. How many bricks can they stack?
9. Can they catch a ball?
10. Can they hop on one leg?
11. Can they run backwards?
12. Can they skip?
13. How do they climb stairs?
14. Can they tell right from left?
15. Can they tie shoe laces?
16. Can they tell you their name and address?
17. Can they write their name?
18. Can they read?
19. Can they add up?
20. Can they recall what presents they had for their birthday?

Fig. 9.2 An observation schedule for use with children at play

Learning to cope with babies poses its own set of problems. With older children, the need to manhandle them is not too frequent since a certain amount of co-operation can be obtained, whereas a baby has to be picked up before anything can be done to it. Ninety per cent of learners have not looked after a baby before and are frightened of doing it wrongly or dropping the baby! Because babies can not only hear but are able to focus their eyes from a very early age, they like to be picked up so they may look round, see human faces and hear voices. Since they even show signs of distress at not hearing a voice when they can see a face, the learner has to be able to talk to them unselfconsciously. As babies cannot talk, the learner has to discover from a cry what the source of discomfort is. In short, she has to learn everything that a mother is supposed to know.

Unfortunately, there is often a dearth of babies on the ward, and anyway a sick baby is not an ideal learning resource. The hospital crèche has been before now (with parental consent) the source of a healthy baby on whom to demonstrate care in class, but the practical answer is to arrange for the learners to do a spell of obstetric experience before being assigned to the paediatric ward.

In recent years, there has been a change in the approach to the nursing of adolescents. It is now becoming usual to look after these youngsters as near as possible to the paediatric ward, and often caring is carried out by the paediatric staff. The clinical teacher must be aware of the difficulties faced by the learner when looking after what can be a volatile age group. Nursing tends to make students mature early, but it is still very easy for them to identify with patients of about their own age. It can be much more of a problem obtaining cooperation from, or when necessary exerting authority over, such patients. Often adolescents may be in the ward for behavioural problems and it then becomes important for the clinical teacher to liaise with the consultant in charge, to enable her to provide support for her learners when dealing with these patients.

A maxim that occasionally crops up in teaching, the truth of which may not be immediately apparent, is that learners remember the point but not the principle. On one occasion during a discussion on pyloric stenosis, a group of students was asked what the doctor would do while the nurse was giving a test feed to the baby. Someone immediately chaffed, 'Stand well back', but then went on to explain that he would palpate the baby's abdomen to feel for a 'tumour', thus running the risk of being in the way if the baby had a projectile vomit. However, some time later in written answers from the same group there appeared the phrase in one reply to the same question 'Stand well back', but with no further explanation. Making a joke about a particular topic can provide a useful peg on which to hang the information; but the teacher must not only supply the information but emphasise it to ensure its retention.

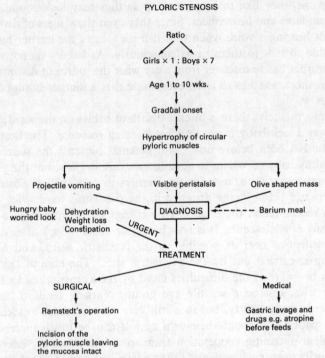

Fig. 9.3 Example of a useful format for teaching hand-outs

Learners like hand-outs' is another aphorism many of us have been taught. What learners do not like are pages of fine typescript. A single page of diagrams or flowcharts, or even a piece of doggerel as an aid to memory, enhances a lecture and is more likely to be used afterwards (Figs. 9.3 and 9.4). If the learner wants a more detailed analysis, then she may make her own notes from the discussion or consult textbooks.

The nursing history sheet and care plan are essential to the nurse working on the paediatric ward (see Fig. 9.5). They provide a complete record of the need for care and the care given to the patient prior to the nurse's allocation or during her days off, and prescribe the further care to be given. When the learner comes to write up a patient care plan herself while caring for a child, she will need the guidance and supervision of the clinical teacher. The care plan becomes a valuable teaching aid and ensures that appropriate care is consistently delivered.

Learners sometimes experience a lot of difficulty in coping with drug calculations. Even if they have A level mathematics, by the time they come to learn paediatrics the ability to work with decimal

To calculate how much of a drug should be administered when the amount required is different from the dose dispensed, the following formula should always be used.

$$\frac{\text{AMOUNT REQUIRED}}{\text{AMOUNT DISPENSED}} \times \text{VOLUME}$$

e.g.

If 10 mgs of a drug is prescribed, and the amount dispensed is 50 mgs in 2 mls, the formula would therefore be:

$$\frac{10}{50} \times 2$$

$$= \frac{20}{50}$$

$$= \frac{2}{5}$$

$$= 0.4 \text{ mls}$$

Now calculate how much you would administer if 6.3 mgs of a drug is prescribed and it is dispensed as 35 mgs in 5 mls . . .

Fig. 9.4 Example of a hand-out for calculation of drug dosages.

points and division has been left far behind. Hence there is a very real need for the clinical teacher to devote some teaching time to the subject, backed by a suitable hand-out as in Fig. 9.4; this allows emphasis on the seriousness of the subject before the learners are allowed on the ward. The subject of digoxin administration forms a basis for such a discussion, since errors made with this drug are frequently fatal.

Safety, while of major concern in any department, becomes of paramount importance on a children's ward. Whereas an adult patient can normally be expected to behave with common sense, mischievous or inquisitive youngsters know no such limits. The student must not only be taught ways of appearing to have eyes in the back of her head, but must also be made to anticipate dangers which might arise and to act to forestall them. A practical approach would be to take a group of students round the ward after telling them to look for potential hazards, and then hold an open discussion on what they noticed, what they should have noticed, and what can be done to prevent such hazards occurring in the first place. Safety is endangered if basic standards of hygiene are not maintained, and nurses should be reminded that parents may well follow examples set by the nursing staff. For example, although pre-packed feeds are frequently used in hospital, a learner may well

3-11 YEARS   Page 1

Surname	SMITH	Date of Admission 14 6 83	Consultant DR. JONES	Medical Diagnosis UNDESCENDED RIGHT TESTICLE
Forenames JOSEPH ANDREW	Address 4 FAIRLAWNS DRIVE BARNET HERTS EN4 8PG		Religion C + E	Baptised – Yes/No
Likes to be referred to as JOEY	Age 5	Date of Birth 3 12 77	Parents C + E	Address OAKHILL PARK HEALTH CENTRE
Hospital No: 58928	Ward	MARY	G.P. DR POSE	OXDPGE LANE BARNET

Next of Kin MRS. S. SMITH **Relationship** MOTHER
Address AS ABOVE

Team Members
Dietitian   Speech Therapist
Occupational Therapist   Physiotherapist
Social Worker   Others

Tel. Nos.: Home 01 – 111 – 1578 **Work**

PERSONAL DATA

Name of person giving history	MRS. S. SMITH	IF NOT PARENTS give reason
By what name is the child called	JOEY	Are there any other children in the family? TWO
Language spoken by parents	ENGLISH	Brothers/Age/Name THOMAS – AGE 8
Language spoken by patient	ENGLISH	Sisters/Age/Name SUZANNE – AGE 3 MONTHS

FOOD/FLUIDS:

Does the child usually have a good appetite	NO	IF NO, what are the problems FUSSY EATER
What type of food does he/she like	CHIPS AND BEANS	
What type of foods does he/she dislike	EGGS AND GREEN VEGETABLES	
What are the child's usual mealtimes at home	8.00 AM 12.30 PM 6.00 PM	
What is the child's favourite drink	LEMONADE COCA COLA TEA	
Is there any drink the child dislikes	WARM MILK	
Does the child prefer drinks hot or cold	VARIES	
Are there any foods the child must not have	EGGS	
Does he/she clean their teeth regularly	YES	
Does the child use a knife and fork	NOT VERY GOOD YET WITH KNIFE	

BED: 4   NAME: JOSEPH SMITH   REL: C + E   CONSULTANT: DR. JONES   HOSP. NO: 58928

Page 2

3-11 YEARS

SLEEP:

What time does he/ go to bed at night	20.20 HRS	What time does he/ awaken in the morning	7.00 HRS
Does the child usually have a drink before he/ goes to bed	NO	Does the child take a favourite toy to bed	YES — "NODDY"

ELIMINATION:

Does he/ have any problems with bowels/passing urine	NO
Does the child ever wet his/ bed	OCCASIONALLY
What words does the child use for bowel action/passing urine	"ONES" and "TWOS"
Does the child use the toilet	YES

RECREATION/EDUCATION:

Does he/• like school	YES — JUST STARTED SCHOOL	IF NO, what is the reason for this
Is he/.. coping with school work	YES	IF NO, what is the reason for this
What does the child like to do in his/ free time	PLAY WITH HIS BROTHER AND READ STORY BOOKS	

STRESS/ENVIRONMENTAL:

Has he/ been in hospital before   YES - FELL & BANGED HIS HEAD (AGED 2½ YRS)
IF YES, how did the child react   QUITE UPSET AT FIRST- MOTHER STAYED WITH HIM
IF YES, did you have any problems when he/ returned home   A FEW SLEEPLESS NIGHTS
Is your child afraid of anything   THE DARK

PARENTS:

Do you wish to be resident   NO   IF NO, will you be able to visit each day and at what times   FROM 09.30 ONWARDS IF ABLE TO BRING BABY
If parents cannot visit each day, give reason why   SMALL BREAST-FED BABY and OLDER CHILD AT SCHOOL
Do you understand why your child is in hospital   NO ONE TO BABY-SIT - FATHER WORKS AWAY   (give parents reason in their own words)   TO HAVE HIS TESTIS PUT INTO HIS SCROTUM

ANY ADDITIONAL INFORMATION:

Girls – have you started your periods	
If YES, do you have any problems	

NURSING ASSESSMENT:

Skin Inspection	CLEAN
Oral Inspection	CLEAN
Condition of hair	CLEAN
General Condition	GOOD
General Observations: Height 110 cm T.P.R. 37° C P 100 R 24
Weight 20.5 Kg Urine N.A.D.

ADDITIONAL OBSERVATIONS:

HISTORY TAKEN BY STUDENT NURSE JEAN BROWN	TIME 11.00 HRS	CONSULTANT: DR JONES	DATE 14.6.83	HOSP. NO: 58928

BED: 4   NAME: JOSEPH SMITH   REL: C & G

Fig. 9.5a Nursing history sheet

DATE COMMENCED	PATIENTS NEEDS/PROBLEM	EXPECTED OUTCOME/PROGRESS	NURSING CARE PLAN	DATE DISCONTINUED
14.6.83	1) Undescended testicle for right orchidopexy.	Admit fully to ward.	Take full nursing history. Assess initial signs.	
	2) Anxiety on admission to hospital.	Alleviate anxiety - a happy stay in hospital.	Introduce to staff and patients. Show around ward and explain procedures. Encourage mother to visit.	
	3) Mother breast-feeding small sister.	Mother to stay as long as possible.	Provide room for mother to breast-feed and facilities to care for small baby.	
	4) Close to older brother.	Maintain contact.	Neighbour to bring brother to hospital after school.	
	5) Occasional enuresis, particularly when stressed.	Try to prevent wet bed.	Take to toilet before bedtime.	
	6) Allergic to eggs.	Prevent ingestion of any egg products.	Do not offer Joey eggs and avoid any products (e.g. cakes) which might contain eggs. Keep an eye on what other children might offer Joey.	
	7) Pre-operative preparation	Prepare Joey physically and mentally for surgery on 15.6.83.	Explain operation to mother and child simply. Ensure Joey understands what is to happen. Repeat explanations p.r.n. Consent form to be signed by mother. Nil by mouth from 6.00 a.m. on 15.6.83. Bath and operation gown. Pre-medication to be given at 9.30 a.m. on 15.6.83. Mother to stay with child during pre-operative period.	

BED: 4   NAME: JOSEPH SMITH   AGE: 5   REL: C.OF.E.   CONSULTANT: DR. JONES   HOSP. NO: 58926

Fig. 9.5b Nursing care plan

find herself being asked by parents for advice on the preparation of feeds. The learner must therefore know and be able to demonstrate the correct way of making them up from first principles.

It is often the case that the responsibility of the clinical teacher lies solely on the wards, and that classroom teaching is outside her province. If, however, the teacher is a specialist in a subject like paediatrics it is of considerable practical advantage to both teacher and learners to integrate classroom and practical teaching as much as possible. Since there can be so many variations on skills, this ensures uniformity of methods with correspondingly fewer chances of confusion on the learner's part. When, for example, the clinical teacher is working with a nurse on the ward, she knows exactly what the learner has been previously taught, so there are no gaps left in the learning nor duplication of effort. Such a system also leads to greater job satisfaction for the teacher, in itself a source of better teaching.

To put this integration into practice, a modular system of training is now usually employed with the clinical teacher, a specialist in her subject, teaching the group of learners for a week in the classroom before working with them on the ward for their clinical allocation, and spending a further week with them at the end of the experience for consolidation in the classroom of what they have learnt. In the general Registration training programme, a paediatric module with a paediatric nurse teacher dealing with both theoretical and practical aspects of her subject would be integrated within the general training pattern. Ideally this should follow an obstetric module in order to give continuity of learning. In the specialist paediatric hospital, each module might be based on the major clinical specialities, e.g. cardiology; or on problems with activities of living. Again the learner would receive teaching in the particular subject in class immediately before dealing with it on the ward.

In the writer's opinion, it is of far greater value if the clinical teacher is attached to one small unit rather than working on a number of wards. She then becomes much more a part of the ward team, as well as becoming accepted by the children and their parents. Acceptance by the children can make the teacher's job so much easier. Although children generally have a trust of nurses instilled into them by parents and books, there was one occasion when the writer, syringe poised, was told by a six year old, 'You can't give me an injection! You're not a nurse, you don't have a hat on!'

When the teacher is attached to a small unit, the learners are more aware of her role and will more readily approach her when, for example, they require help with a particular aspect of care. In addition, the teacher's timetable becomes much more flexible, so she can help many more learners during the course of the day. Doctors also become more willing to request the clinical teacher's help alongside that of a new nurse when carrying out difficult procedures that require special care, for example, holding a child for venepuncture or a lumbar puncture. This means that the learner is taught correctly in the first instance, and the doctor is able to carry out his job in the shortest time, causing least discomfort to the child. The trained ward staff are left to carry out the supervision of nursing care for the other children undisturbed.

Most nurses enjoy working with children. The atmosphere on the ward is of necessity much more relaxed, and nowhere else can one sit on the floor playing with the patients and even singing with them! There are always, though, one or two students in each group who simply do not feel at home with children, and just because the clinical teacher loves infants she should not be unsympathetic to these learners. In fact she should try to help them made the best use of their period of allocation without making life too much of a burden for them.

The clinical teacher in paediatrics may well find herself standing around much more than she would on an adult ward; this is because many paediatric skills only require one person. It takes only one nurse to wash and change a baby, whereas it takes two to do the same to a disabled adult. The teacher is still working in a supervisory capacity, though.

These days, the multi-disciplinary team approach is constantly being advocated as the best way of looking after sick children. With such a system, it becomes essential that the clinical teacher is ward-based rather than school-based. She becomes part of the ward team, not just doing the teaching but encouraging and co-ordinating the other members in passing on their knowledge.

In general, there is no real difference in the teaching techniques used in paediatrics from any other subject. Where the difference lies (particularly on a children's ward in a general hospital) is in the scope of the work. Other wards tend to be more specialised, but the paediatric clinical teacher has to know, and teach learners about, the whole gamut of ailments that affects children. This variety of work is a source of constant satisfaction.

10

Clinical teaching in post-basic education

In the 'good old days', clinical teaching in a specialised unit was a rather haphazard affair. Prior to 1970, all hospitals were free to run courses for staff nurses in any subject that they wished. Many of these courses were excellent, while others were of extremely poor quality: there were no standards of measurement of the quality of the course, apart from those set by the hospital itself; there were no national standards between the courses of either duration or content; there was no guarantee that any educational programme had been pursued, or that the necessary clinical experience and expertise had been achieved by the student. The majority of hospitals issued the students with a certificate on completion of the course; needless to say, this was of little value outside the hospital itself. Many of these courses were being run for the sake of increasing the staffing numbers for the specialist units; the students were therefore being used as 'pairs of hands', especially as in many instances there were no additional finances allocated for the purpose of the course, and it was therefore difficult to release these students to follow any educational programmes.

Following the publishing of a report from the Central Health Service Council in 1966, which highlighted the inadequacies and deficiencies of the existing system, and in conjunction with the findings of a report *Psychiatric Nursing Today* (1968) which recommended post-basic training in psychiatric specialities, the Royal College of Nursing initiated discussions with the Secretary of State. As a result of these discussions, it was agreed that a national body should be set up to rationalise and co-ordinate post basic training in the clinical specialities. This body was to be known as the Joint Board of Clinical Nursing Studies, and it came into being in 1970.

The functions agreed for the Joint Board of Clinical Nursing Studies were to determine which of the clinical specialities required post-basic courses; to assess the manpower needs of each speciality; to lay down national standards for and co-ordinate the planning of

217

such courses; and to award a nationally recognised certificate to all successful students. Since 1983, the functions of the JBCNS have been undertaken by the English and Welsh National Boards for Nursing.

The philosophy of the National Boards is that the overall aim of post-basic clinical education and training is to improve the quality of care given to the patients and to encourage nurses to remain in their particular speciality. This training must be relevant to the job of the nurse in the specialist area; her role must be identified, and it is important that the training is seen by the nurse herself to have relevance and value. The National Boards feel quite strongly that the role of the nurse cannot be considered in isolation; she is part of the team, along with the doctors and other professionals who are involved in meeting the patients' needs (Fig. 10.1).

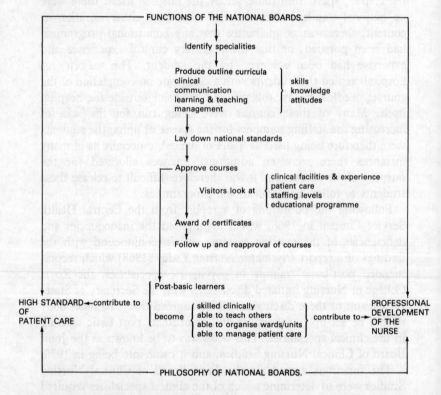

Fig. 10.1 Diagramatic representation of the functions of the National Boards with regard to post basic courses.

When the Joint Board of Clinical Nursing Studies was first set up, it was envisaged that it would be primarily concerned with the needs of nurses and midwives in specialist hospital departments. By 1973, it had extended to such a degree that the community nurses were also included. From its inception the staff of the Joint Board of Clinical Nursing Studies grew considerably. The largest development was that of the Clinical Nursing Studies officers, who were in post throughout the country, ensuring constant contact between the Joint Board of Clinical Nursing Studies with its policy making function and the service itself. This channel of communication is now maintained by the National Boards' Education Officers for continuing education and training.

Doctors and nurses who are experts in the particular specialty form the National Boards' panels, which advise on matters relating to each course; and this pattern is repeated in the team which sets up courses in individual centres. Each panel has within its terms of reference the functions of:

planning the outline curricula
defining the course objectives
determining the length of the course
setting the criteria for entry.

As well as setting up full time post-basic courses, the National Boards also institute short courses to interest the more experienced staff; these offer them the opportunity to study an aspect of the clinical subject that is related to the work that they are currently involved in. These short courses are also based on a national curriculum, prepared by specialist panels and a statement of attendance is given on completion.

The outline curricula are prepared in such a way that they ensure that the training encompasses the needs of the patients in that particular speciality; they also ensure that the programme is flexible enough to adapt to the changing techniques and advances in technology. Initially, this method of curriculum design was unfamiliar to the nurses involved in running and setting up individual courses; for this reason, a series of workshops was held in different parts of the country. When drawing up the outline curricula, the panel of specialists first establishes the aim of the course; for example, the aim of the Renal Nursing course is 'to train registered nurses in the special aspects of nursing patients with renal disease and those undergoing dialysis and renal transplantation'. The objectives of the course are then defined; these state in broad terms what the nurse should be able to perform on completion of the course. This detailed definition of the specific objectives clarifies for the learner the learning opportunities that are available. The objectives are broken down into skills, knowledge and attitudes (Table 10.1).

The term 'skill' refers not only to manual dexterity but also to competence in communication, management and research. All students are advised to obtain a copy of the outline curriculum before commencing a course, so that they will know exactly the standard they should be able to achieve during the training.

Table 10.1

Objectives 3
At the end of the course the nurse will have knowledge of, and interest in, basic teaching methods

Skills	*Knowledge*	*Attitudes*
Application of teaching methods to the staff, patients and their relatives.	Introduction to principles and methods of learning, teaching and testing.	Appreciate the importance of teaching others and is willing to accept this responsibility.
	Special problems of teaching patients and relatives.	

From the outline curriculum. *Renal Nursing*. Course Number 136.

The initiative to set up a post-basic course comes from either the Health Authority or the Nurse Education Centre of the hospital concerned. In planning the distribution of courses, the National Boards take into account such factors as population, the availability of clinical experience, nursing manpower in the particular clinical area, recruitment for existing courses, and the likelihood of job vacancies for students on completion of the course.

It is felt that in order to establish and maintain a national standard, all courses should be planned and run on educational principles; any centre wishing to run a specialist course must therefore first examine their educational and clinical facilities, and if necessary look into the possibility of combining with another centre. The financial implications of running a course must be identified, taking into account salaries and expenses of staff and students, lecture fees, teaching equipment and books.

The National Boards suggest the appointment of a nurse teacher in the Education division with responsibility for post-basic education together with a specialist clinical teacher for each course. It is further recommended that the number of students be related to the clinical experience available, the number of other staff in the clinical area and the number of trained staff available to provide supervision and teaching.

The planning team, which consists of representatives from the tutorial and medical staff and other professional groups involved with the speciality, can contact their Regional Educational Officers for informal advice and suggestions at any time. As the planning team is multidisciplinary, there is an increasing awareness of the totality of patient care, and an increasing involvement of these disciplines with one another.

Once the completed application form and a copy of the suggested course programme have been received by the National Boards, the centre receives a visit from the specialist team. During this visit, which usually occupies one or two days, the team meets members of the planning team, visits the clinical areas involved, and holds discussions with members of staff, both medical and nursing. The school of nursing and other teaching facilities are inspected, and the educational programme is discussed with the tutorial staff. Following this visit, the Education Officer presents an official report to the Applications Committee, who may require further information or suggest modifications to be made before approval is given. Approval is given for a stated number of courses and a maximum number of students.

When an approved course has been running for some time, it will receive a visit from the Education Officer to ascertain that changes are being instituted in accordance with end of course evaluation sessions, and to make recommendations for improvements. Any changes which affect the course, either in local conditions or because of suggestions made at evaluation, must be notified to the National Board. The Education Officer may visit the centre to assess the effect of these changes. When approval is required, the Officer may also visit, before a request is considered. Application for reapproval must be submitted at least six months in advance.

The National Boards issue circulars stating any changes in policy. These, along with a list of approved post-basic courses, are sent to the schools of nursing. Various booklets were produced by the Joint Board to help tutors and clinical teachers running the courses; an example of one of these is 'The Management objective in Joint Board outline curricula' (1980). This booklet was prepared 'to help tutors plan the management objective of the outline curricula and to suggest what should feature in the detailed teaching programme.'

Meetings and study days for teachers are held by the National Boards. Topics related to post-basic education (e.g. methods of assessment, evaluation, formulating objectives) are discussed and guidance given as necessary. These meetings have proved to be particularly helpful, allowing teachers the opportunity to discuss mutual problems and to exchange ideas.

The Joint Board recognised the advantage of internally controlled assessments, as opposed to a national examination. Continuous assessment of students is encouraged by the National Boards. Research staff at the Joint Board were responsible for examining such aspects as the assessment of courses, carrying out surveys, finding out what nurses do on completion of their courses, and whether or not they have found their training valuable. Unfortunately the National Boards have been unable to undertake this commitment.

The responsibility of the clinical teacher in post-basic education is two-fold. She must have a detailed knowledge of the particular specialty and be capable of teaching the associated skills in the clinical area. She is also involved, together with the Senior Nurse Tutor, in planning the education programme and in classroom teaching during study periods. Students come from many different backgrounds and present a variety of experience. Some may experience difficulty in adjusting to a new environment and the challenge of the course. It is here that the Clinical Teacher must play a helpful and supportive role, counselling when necessary and generally establishing rapport with the students.

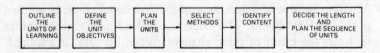

Fig. 10.2 Order in which the outline curriculum can be translated into a detailed curriculum

Planning and arranging the programme (Fig. 10.2)

The programme is planned, using the National Board's outline curriculum as a guide; this states the units of learning to be included and the objectives to be achieved by the student, defined and broken down into the relevant skills, knowledge and attributes. Each unit can be further divided into smaller, more manageable units. Periods of study can then be devoted to one skill, or a group of skills that are inter-related either to one another or to an aspect of patient care.

Selecting the methods of learning to be used and identifying the content go very much hand in hand; there are obviously many ways in which the nurse can be helped to master the skills that are specified in the objectives. The methods selected will depend entirely on many factors, e.g. the availability of equipment and facilities, and the skills to be learned. The clinical teacher will also know from previous experience which methods have been successful.

The time allocated to each unit of learning will depend on the amount of theoretical and clinical experience underlying each skill, the opportunities that are available to practice the skill, and the importance of that skill in relation to others that are to be learned. It is important that these units of learning are placed in the programme in a logical, meaningful sequence, so that the students are not learning to run before they can walk. The programme should be arranged in such a way that it provides a framework of knowledge covering all the different physiological, pathological, nursing and social aspects, so that the learner has the understanding necessary to apply this knowledge in a given situation. Ideally the clinical experience should occur in conjunction with the appropriate unit of learning. Inter-related units of learning should be taught in conjunction with one another, so that the students can integrate them and consolidate their learning. The students will need time in the clinical area to practise and become proficient in these skills, so that at the end of their course they are safe and efficient practitioners.

When planning the course, flexible scheduling is important wherever possible, so that the levels of ability of the individual students can be catered for, and they can progress at their own rate. It may be necessary to be flexible about group size and the teaching environment, so that modified lectures, discussion groups, tutorials, seminars and study periods can all be used to provide variations in teaching. Individual tuition is usually easy to arrange as the majority of post-basic courses have a clinical teacher/student ratio of approximately 1:6. It may be necessary in some cases to adjust the amount of time that individual students remain in certain clinical areas, so that they can become proficient at certain skills in their own time; those who master these skills easily can be moved to a new area, so that they do not become bored and lose their motivation, while those who are somewhat slower do not become pressurised and anxious.

All members of the team involved with patient care in the specialised area can contribute considerably to the teaching of students, and their cooperation is essential. Including them in the programme, and asking for advice and suggestions regarding the planning of the programme creates greater interest and co-operation from these other staff members. The learners should also be encouraged to take an interest in the day-to-day planning of the programme, by finding out for themselves where specialised procedures are being carried out elsewhere in the hospital, so that arrangements can be made for them to observe these.

A pre-test given at the beginning of the course helps to identify individual learning needs. Objective type questions can be used for this; they provide a wide content coverage, and pose a series of precise problems which can be clearly stated and can be accurately marked. The information acquired from this can be used to adjust the amount and depth of teaching, identify individual needs, and locate strengths and weaknesses that should be taken into account when helping a student to progress. Knowledge should be pre-tested at the beginning of each unit of learning and post-tested at the beginning of each unit of learning and post-tested before the next unit.

Evaluation is an integral part of an approved post-basic course, and it is planned at the outset with other details of the programme. The National Boards recommend that a day is set aside towards the end of the course to determine whether the course as a whole has achieved its aims and objectives. Students, together with educational and clinical staff, have an opportunity to review and discuss the course and make suggestions for change. All reasonable suggestions are properly considered, discussed at planning team meetings and implemented, if appropriate.

Any changes that are implemented following these meetings will have been properly considered.

The Joint Board issued an excellent evaluation package which consists of forms to be used by:
– the planning team to evaluate the efficiency of their performance
– the students to evaluate the course
– the teacher to evaluate her own teaching
– the students to evaluate the teaching methods.

Running the course

The purpose of the course is to enable the learner to achieve the course objectives. The student's progress is monitored and assessed continuously, both practically and theoretically. This helps to ensure that the student has achieved the broad objectives as outlined in the curriculum, and the detailed objectives set by the centre. All objectives are stated in behavioural terms, making it clear exactly what the student will be able to achieve in a given time.

The National Boards have the responsibility for establishing and maintaining courses on a national basis and with a minimum national standard; while recognising the difficulty of maintaining this standard, the Boards believe that there are certain factors which should help in its achievement, one of which is valid and reliable assessments. The centre decides the average mark which must be achieved by the student in written assessments, and this is explained at interview and at the beginning of the course.

The courses themselves can be extremely intensive and it is therefore more logical to monitor the student's progress through each objective of the course. This can be achieved effectively by arranging for the learner to undertake practical assessments in all clinical areas; for appraisals to be carried out by senior nursing members in the clinical areas; for the individual student to submit or present nursing care studies and a research project; and to set both the written and multiple choice type paper following each session of study in the school of nursing.

The marks for each of these can go towards the student's final grade. In this way, it is possible to pin-point the areas where the student requires additional guidance and advice, and to act upon this immediately.

The learners undertaking a post-basic course come to the course with a varied range of nursing experience and knowledge of the world and its problems; their reasons for pursuing this particular course will range from a desire to increase their knowledge, to personal, professional and occupational goals.

There will also be those who are 'collecting certificates' because they cannot decide which way to go. Those learners who have come from schools of nursing with traditional learning backgrounds, and those who have not been studying for some time, may find it difficult to accept responsibility for their own learning and to adjust to the more individualised tuition. The clinical teacher must there-fore (especially during the first few months of the course) play a helpful and supportive role; she should try to establish rapport with her students, so that they feel that she is available to help them.

The learners will need a thorough orientation to what the course involves, and how the specialist unit expects them to function as members of the team. They should be given a framework for the entire course, with the total time allotted for specific clinical areas, study days, holidays, the dates of examinations and when individual nursing care studies and research projects are to be completed. They also should be given a National Board outline curriculum, so that they are aware of the specific aims and objectives of the course they have undertaken and the skills that are to be pursued and learned.

As many of the learners will be new to the hospital, a thorough introduction to the hospital, its personnel, policies and practices is very important. Without this, a feeling of insecurity and loneliness may add to the other difficulties of adjustment in an entirely new and strange situation. Informal meetings with the staff in the specialist unit and practical sessions in the clinical area, rather than in the classroom during the initial orientation week, will make the learners less nervous when they first venture into these areas.

The clinical teacher needs to be constantly in the clinical area with her students during their first few months; this will be less necessary towards the end of the course, as they become more confident, able and less in need of support.

The clinical teacher should initially help the students to plan and organise their daily assignments, and to apply their newly acquired knowledge in the clinical field. She should assist them in the development of their observational and management skills, and make suggestions for their patients' care; as the students progress, she should gradually leave them more on their own, giving them a chance to assume more responsibility for the planning and implementation of care for the patient. As the learners gain expertise and proficiency, group or individual meetings can be held daily to discuss the learners' proposed nursing care plans, and to guide them as necessary. Each revision that is made provides good learning opportunities. At the end of the day, a similar session can be held to evaluate the care that the patient has received and to make suggestions for further revisions.

The clinical teacher should circulate among all of her students, allowing time to help all of them, rather than helping a few at the expense of others. This can be difficult if the learners are working in widely distributed clinical areas in the hospital. The clinical teacher must therefore arrange her programme to cover this eventuality. She should always allow for unexpected changes in the learning programme, and be aware of other resources that are available; she must have a good rapport with all other staff members, so that when specialised procedures of interest to course members are being carried out they ensure that she is informed, and arrangements can be made for the learners to be present.

The learners should be encouraged to take advantage of all the learning opportunities and resources that are available – not just to use the library, but also to read their patients' medical histories, participate in doctors' ward rounds, visit the out-patients' clinics, and ask questions.

The advent of the Nursing Process has added a new dimension to post-basic education, and the clinical teacher can introduce the concept to the students and give guidance on its implementation. Informal teaching sessions, either on a one-to-one basis, or with course members, where the patient's problems are discussed, are valuable and guidance can be given on effective methods of communication with patients and staff.

One of the objectives to be achieved by learners undertaking an approved post-basic course is that the nurse should be able to apply the skills and knowledge that she has acquired and impart them effectively to patients, relatives and staff.

The learners should be encouraged to work with the student nurses at every available opportunity, so that they can teach them about the specialised procedures that are being carried out and the principles behind them. If the course members are preparing nursing care studies, it is useful if they can take an aspect of this, and present it to their peer group as a teaching topic. If this is carried out as an informal session, all course members begin to learn how to overcome the embarrassment of imparting information when teaching. This also prepares them for presenting their research project at the end of the course.

Included in the final objective for all courses approved by the National Boards is that the nurses should have an appreciation of research. Ideally, a member of the school of nursing staff, or an outside speaker with experience in the field of research, should speak to the course members. Unfortunately this is not always possible, so the clinical teacher must be prepared to teach on this topic. Using the Joint Board of Clinical Nursing Studies booklet (1977) 'Research Objectives in Joint Board Courses', the clinical teacher can draw up a written guide for the learners to help them to choose a subject to research; collect data; analyse the information; and draw conclusions from this information. Initially, the learners will be full of enthusiasm to research the most enormous subject; gradually, as they realise the task that they have set themselves, they will choose something more realistic. The smaller and more useful projects would seem to be the most successful. The hardest job for the clinical teacher during this phase is not to prepare the entire project for the learners; unless carefully briefed, however, they will send out far more questionnaires than they need, with ambiguously worded questions, so that just before they are due to report their findings there is complete confusion. By the time that they have reached the stage of the course when they are preparing their research project, the majority of the learners have regained their confidence in their ability to cope, so that the clinical teacher must be tactful in her approach and offers of help and guidance.

Another aspect of the final objective in the outline curriculum is that the learner will have an understanding of the management and organisation of the ward, unit or department. In many instances, this objective is misread and the learners may come to the clinical teacher very concerned because they do not feel that they are capable of running the specialised area at the end of their course. The key word in this objective is 'understanding'; it is not envisaged that students will be skilled at the end of the course, in this respect. There may be nurses of exceptional ability who can spend half of their time in the lecture room, a quarter in the clinical area and the other quarter in other departments, and still at the end of the course be able to manage and organise the unit. But this will not necessarily be so. As these specialised courses place as much emphasis on theoretical knowledge as on practical skills, the majority of learners really require at least three months after they have completed the course to consolidate their learning. One way to help them gain an understanding of the management and organisation involved is to arrange with the senior members of staff that the learners run the specialised areas on occasions with supervision. The senior member of staff or clinical teacher should be present for support during the early days, but as learners gain confidence in their own ability they should gradually manage the unit on their own under all circumstances.

As the course progresses, the students will need time to put into practice the skills that they have learned. The clinical teacher should leave them to master these skills at their own pace; those who have acquired this mastery should be encouraged to pursue independent study projects of particular interest, not necessarily part of the formal course objectives, but designed to contribute additional knowledge and understanding. During this period, the clinical teacher together with the planning team must start evaluating for herself the success and future of the course and identify those aspects that need to be altered for the next intake, and can begin to plan the programme for the subsequent course.

Post-basic courses make several demands on the health service. The financial commitment itself is quite large; the learners may only be spending four days a week in the clinical environment, the remainder of their time being spent in the classroom. The relevant clinical experience may not be readily available, and it may be necessary to send the students elsewhere to gain this. Without the co-operation of the ward staff, it is not possible for course members to study in the wards or to have the opportunities to observe practical procedures, read patients' notes or to partake in doctors' ward rounds; it is therefore vital that the ward staff are encouraged to feel that they can contribute to the running and management of the course. The advantages of these courses to the Health Service are many: recruitment to the specialist units is improved, the retention in the specialized clinical units of course members following completion of their course is invaluable; the enthusiasm and interest of the course members is contagious, and non-course members gain knowledge alongside them. These learners bring a highly developed enquiring attitude to clinical practice. The nursing care studies and research projects that are carried out by the course members provide valuable information, and because of these factors the standard of nursing care is greatly improved among all members of staff. For the clinical teacher running a post-basic course, these factors have a large bearing on the overall approach to the course; enthusiasm on the part of the clinical teacher and confidence in her course members' ability to succeed will increase the enthusiasm and interest of the course members. The relationships that the clinical teacher establishes with her students, peers, nursing staff in the clinical area and staff in related health and welfare departments, will affect the efficiency of the running and organisation of the entire course. The prevailing atmosphere in the clinical setting and the professional example set by the clinical teacher is a vital factor in setting the learning pace in the clinical environment; the learners must feel that they can approach the clinical teacher at all times; the clinical teacher must motivate and encourage her students, and at all times maintain a climate that is conducive to learning.

The ultimate goal of both the specialised unit and the school of nursing is to provide the optimum in patient care. Since 1970, thanks to the Joint Board of Clinical Nursing Studies, this has become more of a reality than it was previously; as the clinical teacher running an approved post basic course, in close proximity to patients, learners, and ward staff, and with the facilities of the school of nursing to use, one is in an excellent position to help in achieving this goal.

Acknowledgement

I would like to thank Miss M. G. Gardener O.B.E., S.R.N., S.C.M., R.N.T., N.A. (H) Cert., for her kind permission to quote from the literature published by the Joint Board of Clinical Nursing Studies.

REFERENCES

The Joint Board of Clinical Nursing Studies (1977) *The Research Objective in Joint Board Courses, An Introductory Guide.* Occasional Publications, Kingston Printers.
The Joint Board of Clinical Nursing Studies (1980) *The Managment Objective in Joint Board Outline Curricula.* Occasional Publications, Kingston Printers.
Ministry of Health, Central Health Services Council (1968) *Psychiatric Nursing Today and Tomorrow.* London: Her Majesty's Stationery Office.
Standing Nursing Advisory Committee of the Central Health Council (1966) *The Post Certificate Training and Education of Nurses.* London: Her Majesty's Stationery Office.

11

The developing role of the teacher in the clinical sphere

Teachers in the clinical sphere include all those trained nurses who help students in hospital or the community to learn from their clinical nursing experience. The role of these teachers should not be considered in isolation since roles develop in response to changing demands. Social changes which affect the work setting, whether this be in hospital or in the patients' homes, developments in nursing practice and education all contribute to shaping and modifying the role of teachers in the clinical sphere. Developments influencing the setting in which all of these teachers function will be examined before focussing on the role of the teachers themselves.

The changing social scene

Nursing is concerned with helping people to live full and happy lives, free if possible from the constraints imposed by disease, handicap or disability or, if this is impossible, helping to provide the support required to enable them to live successfully despite disability or ill-health. Hence it is concerned with living and life-styles. Notions of what constitutes a good life are dependent on peoples' values and expectations, which in turn are influenced by circumstances since these largely determine the availability of choices and opportunities.

Consider, for example, the increased choices and opportunities provided by advances in science and technology. What an impact the availability of man-made fibres has had on the lives of house-wives! Easy to launder and maintain, hard wearing and relatively cheap compared with natural fibres, these materials have also freed her from the hard labour of complicated ironing. Labour-saving devices such as vacuum cleaners, washing machines and tumble dryers have made it possible for career women to work and maintain a home without undue fatigue. Radio and television have given people access to information, ideas and opinions which help to shape attitudes, values and perceptions, as do the increased opportunities for travel provided by modern transport systems.

Nursing and nursing education always have to be considered within the relevant social context. It is a mistake to criticise the practices of former years without bearing in mind the opportunities and constraints of that particular time. It is equally mistaken to look back longingly to systems and practices which worked well years ago, and to complain that standards are falling, without recognising that traditional practice requires constant modification to take account of present circumstances.

It is impossible to consider in detail the influence of social change on all fields of nursing or to examine all the factors contributing to social change throughout this century. Therefore, the subject will be considered with referrence to two settings – one a hospital ward in the 1930s, the other a present-day hospital ward. The background, material circumstances and, insofar as these are relevant to health care, the attitudes, beliefs and perceptions of the patients and staff in these wards will be outlined and any differences noted. It is as well to recognise that there are limitations to this approach. For instance, gaps are left which require bridging by further reading, and the descriptions of each setting are somewhat artificial since ward populations are never quite typical of their day.

A women's ward in a general hospital in the 1930s

Imagine that you have just entered the ward from the main hospital corridor. It is an open ward of the Nightingale type and it is possible to observe all the patients from the door leading to the ward itself. The first thing that might strike you is that all the patients are in bed and that they are all wearing plain, homely nightdresses which are, in fact, hospital issue. The ward is very clean, the furniture and floor are highly polished and there is an absence of clutter. The patients who are well enough to take an interest in their surroundings may be reading or chatting to each other or just observing the scene. There are of course no headphones or television.

You will observe that the vast majority – perhaps all – of the patients are natives of the British Isles, and if you converse with them you will discover that probably none have ever been abroad. Indeed some may never have travelled more than a few miles from their home. Most of these patients left school at the age of fourteen.

You might see a patient admitted. She probably has no toilet equipment, nightdress, dressing gown or slippers. The condition of the patient's clothing will depend on her circumstances and upbringing. She might have gone to great lengths to procure decent underwear for her visit to hospital, the family rallying around to ensure that she is properly equipped, for some of these patients are very self-respecting. Another patient, equally proud but in less favourable circumstances, will have seen that her well-worn clothes are clean and mended. Some patients come as they are. A fair proportion of these patients are badly housed and lack those facilities which encourage attention to personal hygiene. You will gather from these observations that poverty is common. Some of the patients look undernourished and exhausted – indeed many are extremely deprived. Unemployment rates are high and some of the married women work to help to maintain the family. On the whole, however, it is not considered suitable for married women to go out to work; men are seen as the breadwinners and women as the home-makers. In fact, men tend to see themselves as failures if their wives have to work to supplement the family income. Married women are certainly not expected to have a career of their own; the majority of those who do work take unskilled jobs in factories or as domestics in institutions or offices. Most of the unmarried patients also hold relatively lowly posts in offices, shops or factories – it is unusual to find a professional woman among the patients.

The patients are generally uninformed about their illnesses or treatment. You may find one or two 'regulars' who know about hospital routine, perhaps understanding a little about medical and nursing care from their own experience and being more than ready to pass on their knowledge to apprehensive newcomers. The majority, however, are prepared to accept treatment unquestioningly – at least it appears so. Generally they do not have sufficient knowledge, confidence or an adequate vocabulary to discuss their treatment or to question advice. They may perhaps make comments to each other such as 'Well, you are in their hands!', 'They never tell you anything!' or 'they are very clever here, they know what they are doing.' Some of the patients might comment on the comfort the hospital provides, good food, warmth and above all, rest. Those patients who come from comfortable homes are rather less favourably impressed, but for many hospital is a haven – even though the rules might be irksome and their illness a cause of anxiety. There are, of course other anxieties. For instance, some women are worried because their husbands are unable to contrive and scrape as they have learned to do in managing the household budget and debts are accumulating. They are able to discuss their problems with their husbands or other relatives or friends when they visit. Visitors are allowed to come for half-an-hour on most evenings and for one or two hours on Saturday and Sunday afternoons. Some of these patients will be in hospital for several weeks, and worry about losing contact with their young children, but children are never allowed to visit.

The nursing staff. The nursing staff comprises the ward sister, a deputy sister, a staff nurse and five probationer nurses. The latter are at various stages of training and all are preparing for registration. All the staff are natives of the British Isles including four from Eire (as it is now). Their social and educational backgrounds are somewhat varied. The staff nurse comes from a relatively affluent family and attended a private school as a boarder. She has no educational certificates. The deputy sister and two of the probationers 'passed the scholarship' (later known as the eleven plus), and they were all fortunate in being able to accept places at the high school. Two, including the deputy sister gained the School Certificate, but one had to leave before taking the examination due to family misfortune, her father losing his job. Two of the Irish probationers were educated at convent schools until the age of sixteen, obtaining a leaving certificate. The ward sister, who is Irish, and the remaining probationer were educated in convent schools until the age of fourteen, their families being unable to support them beyond that time. The ward sister filled in the gap between school and her entry into nurse training by working as a nanny, the probationer worked as a shop assistant. All the nurses are unmarried and all live in the nurses' home.

The nurses work long hours for a low salary. They themselves expect to do so and society expects them to do so too. Nurses have a vocation; their work is considered to be worthwhile and satisfying although all expect it to be demanding. Possibly, though, not all do have a vocation and resent having to work so very hard for so little material reward.

The probationers. There is certainly a good deal of drudgery as well as interest in the probationers' daily routine. They help with domestic work such as sweeping the ward when the maid is off-duty, washing up, dusting, cleaning equipment and polishing locker tops. The have to work speedily to get through their allotted tasks, and they may be criticised harshly if their work is not up to standard. Discipline is strict, and they are not expected to question or protest when asked to do something. (Some do, of course.) Nevertheless there are bright spots. Cleaning equipment in the sluice can provide an escape from the emotional strains of patient care, cleaning lockers provides an excellent opportunity for getting to know the patients and, as always, patient contact is very rewarding. Long hours, together with longer patient stay in hospital, provide opportunities for continuity of observation and care and the development of closer nurse/patient relationships. When the nurses do get off duty, they do not have to struggle home through the milling crowds and, although they are dependent on the provisions made for their comfort by the hospital authorities, at least they do not have to set about housework and cooking at the end of a day's work at the hospital.

The public believes nurses to be rather noble, giving up much for the good of humanity. Nurses, for the most part, are held in high regard, and the needy often consult them on matters concerning health care. In hospital, the hierarchical structure is very marked; even the probationer who started training one month previously is very much a senior colleague and regards herself as such. Some nurses are unduly aware of their position of authority and are aloof and unapproachable – the patients do not usually complain but may discuss these individuals in an uncomplimentary way, warning newcomers that they 'should take no notice' and 'should not ask *her* for anything.'

The probationers usually attend lectures during their off-duty. The programme of theoretical instruction is limited, but some of the lectures given by senior members of the medical staff are excellent and enjoyed by those who are not too tired to profit from them. There is very little evidence of an attempt to correlate theoretical instruction with practical experience.

Unless the nurses have private means their off-duty activities have to be tailored in accordance with their modest salaries. The communal life in the nurses' home encourages the development of friendships between probationers of the same seniority. Social activities organised for hospital staff are usually well-attended, the dances providing opportunities for meeting members of the opposite sex. Complimentary tickets for theatres or concerts are occasionally available and many nurses spend some of their off-duty at the cinema, which is very popular. Despite strict rules designed to prevent fraternisation, nurses in teaching hospitals meet – and some eventually marry – medical students. Rules in the nurses' home are very strict. Probationers are expected to be in the home, and indeed in their rooms, by a certain time, perhaps 10.30 p.m. They have to report in, and if they are late must explain why and possibly be reprimanded. Probationers are allowed to sleep out for a limited number of nights per month, must give notice of their intention of doing so and, again, are expected to report back. These rules give some indication of society's attitudes: young women have to be protected from moral danger, and, in the case of probationers, from fatigue resulting from too many late nights which would render them unfit for their arduous work. The hospital authorities act *in loco parentis* in the persons of the matron and the home sister, who is directly responsible for discipline in the nurses' home.

Holidays may be spent at home with the family or with friends. Some enterprising probationers may travel around the country on cheap hostelling holidays, but few have the means to take holidays abroad. Following registration, quite a number of nurses leave to get married and those who stay on may be required to do a staff year in order to obtain their hospital certificate and badge. Nurses from general hospitals often consider their training incomplete unless they qualify as midwives, indeed this qualification is essential in order to broaden their career prospects. There are opportunities for working overseas, perhaps in the Colonial Nursing Service, and some are called to work as missionaries. They can, of course, opt to continue with hospital nursing in this country, probably as ward sisters when they have gained sufficient experience, or to train as district nurses, health visitors or industrial nurses.

The ward sister. She is, perhaps, in her early thirties and has been a ward sister for three years. Before being appointed as sister in charge of the ward, she has had experience as a staff nurse, a relief sister and a night sister, during which time she has had the opportunity to learn a good deal from observing her senior colleagues' methods of ward administration. She is directly responsible to the matron for the standard of care in the ward. This entails responsibility for 'ward housekeeping' and the supervision of the work of the domestic staff as well as the actual nursing. She has had no formal preparation for this work; experience is considered to be all important in enabling her to fulfil her functions effectively.

She plans care and allocates duties to nursing and domestic staff, and there is a well organised routine in this ward. She is an exacting person and a recognised authority figure, she knows her job and expects her staff to follow her instructions to the letter. For instance, sister does a ward round with the night nurse, checking that all is in order. If later she discovers something amiss, the night nurse may be called back to give an account of herself and, if sister thinks necessary, to be reprimanded and required to put the matter right. Sister is concerned for the well-being of the patients, she knows them well and they have confidence in her but some may also be slightly in awe of her. She usually takes the opportunity to work with a probationer when performing treatments or giving care to very sick patients. She usually likes to arrange the flowers, the pleasant finishing touch to the appearance of the ward, and observes all that is going on as she undertakes this task. She serves the patients' meals, taking each patient's needs and preferences into account and seeing that the nurses check that the food is acceptable to the patient. If not, she will direct and supervise the preparation of some light delicacy more suited to a jaded appetite. She is, in fact, something of a mother figure; a home-maker as well as a person with special knowledge and skills.

One consultant has beds in her ward and, except when she is on holiday, she is always available to do the regular ward rounds with him. The consultant's role is well defined. He is responsible for directing the treatment of the patients; sister supports and facilitates the implementation of this treatment, and generally what the consultant says goes because he knows best what is needed. In this ward the sister/consultant relationship is a happy one, because the consultant is not only well-informed and skilled but also respects and shows his appreciation of the ward sister's competence, recognising the importance of skilled nursing care. The relationship is less happy in wards where either the consultant is over-bearing or unappreciative, or where the ward sister is less competent or caring or perhaps is too diffident to express herself effectively. The consultant's ward rounds are major events. Everything is carefully prepared and organised down to the new tablet of soap and the newly laundered hand towel. The round tends to be a ceremonious occasion, the ritual giving emphasis to the prestige and importance of the consultant, thus helping to foster confidence in his wisdom. Sister helps and guides new housemen to work in harmony with the consultant and they usually rely on her very much for information and advice about the management of the patients' treatment. (Incidentally, it is this type of ward sister to whom some of the present day senior medical staff refer with such respect and regard. These sisters were indeed the salt of the earth, meeting the needs of their era with great efficiency and dedication.)

There are a few opportunities for professional development. For instance, sister could study for the Diploma in Nursing which is considered to be a worthwhile qualification for nurse practitioners and teachers. If she is especially interested in administration she might consider studying for the Housekeeping Certificate.

A women's ward in a general hospital in the 1980s

Imagine that this is a ward in a modern District General Hospital. The approach to the ward is through a spacious waiting area for visitors furnished with durable but brightly upholstered chairs. There is a wide corridor leading to the ward itself, off which one can observe a day room where several patients are watching television. The ward is sectioned forming bays accommodating four or six patients; there are also several single rooms. A few patients are wandering around the ward; one is supporting a urine drainage bag as she makes her way to the bathroom, others are stopping to talk to bed patients. Several of the patients who are in bed are receiving intravenous infusions and two nurses are adjusting the position of one of these patients. Some of the patients are wearing headphones listening to the radio, one is using the telephone trolley to make a call. The physiotherapist is helping a patient to walk, a laboratory technician is taking a blood specimen, one doctor is writing up notes, another is taking a history from one of the patients. Three patients have visitors, and a porter is taking a patient in a wheelchair to the X-ray department. Two nurses are doing a drug round, and sister is at the nurses' station talking to the dietitian. It is difficult to see all that is happening as one enters the ward, because so many activities are in progress and, in any case, some parts of the ward are not directly observable from the entrance.

The patients. They come from varied backgrounds. Whilst most in this ward are natives of the British Isles, there is a lady from Trinidad, one from Pakistan, a Danish au pair girl and a visitor from Canada who is working temporarily in this country. Most of those from the British Isles have been abroad for holidays, mainly to Europe, but one has visited her daughter in the United States whilst another has just returned from Nigeria where her husband has been working with a United Nations organisation. Their standard of education ranges from that of some of the older patients who left school at fourteen years to that of the Canadian patient who is a graduate in psychology. The younger patients from this country have been educated until at least the age of fifteen and some have achieved several passes in the General Certificate of Education.

Generally these patients appear to be affluent compared with those of the 1930s. All, except one old lady, are wearing their own nightdresses of varied colour and style. Most possess attractive dressing gowns and slippers, and lockers are well equipped with toilet articles including spray perfumes and talcum powder. They do not look undernourished, indeed some are overweight. However, even in this small group, one patient, the old lady, is obviously rather deprived; poverty and poor housing have by no means been completely eliminated. Most of these women work, including the married ones who may have either a full-time or a part-time job. The lady who had just returned from Nigeria is a dietitian, the Trinidadian patient is an Enrolled Nurse from another hospital, there is in the group a secondary school teacher, a catering manageress, a personal assistant to a business executive and an air hostess. The remaining patients work in offices, shops or factories with the exception of the lady from Pakistan, the older patient who has completed a life's work in office cleaning and two middle aged ladies who do voluntary work rather than paid employment. It is noteworthy that attitudes to married women taking a job have changed. The second world war helped to change people's perceptions of the role of married women. So many worked to help the war effort, discovered a new independence and welcomed the opportunity to supplement the family income, that it gradually became acceptable for married women to work, especially after their children started school. Most consider they work from necessity, but notions of necessity often involve maintaining a home furnished with modern equipment and amenities. Expectations have changed; the standard of living which so many of their mothers accepted as normal would not be considered at all adequate. Advertising has helped to encourage people to seek and obtain greater comfort and convenience in the home. Wants have become needs and every facility and encouragement are provided for meeting these new needs through hire purchase and 'do-it-yourself'. Not all are capable of achieving the generally improved standard of living for various reasons, including lack of ability or skill, lack of motivation, perhaps stemming from deprivation of a secure family environment, or lack of strength due to age or disability. Some still live in appalling conditions and are disadvantaged in every way. Those who do strive for better living standards may find it an effort to keep abreast of financial commitments, and stressful to hold down a job and make a home for the family. However, husbands, particularly the younger ones, tend to do more to help with the care of children and household chores.

These patients, who on the whole are used to comfort, plentiful food and reasonably pleasant surroundings tend to be more discerning and even critical of hospital standards. Patients from other cultures may feel that they have grounds for complaint for another sort of reason, that is if staff are unaware or insensitive to their special needs e.g. dietary restrictions.

Most of these patients are fairly well-informed about hospital life and medical treatment. Some have received at least as good a general education as the staff, and are well equipped to seek explanations or challenge decisions. Others with a more limited education have obtained their information through the media, particularly from watching television programmes and reading simplified accounts of medical disorders and their treatment in popular magazines. These patients may need more help than the completely uninformed, who are more likely to leave everything to the experts, whilst the partially informed know enough to worry but not quite enough to understand. This sometimes results in unreasonable demands, misunderstanding and aggressiveness. On the other hand, quite a number of patients even now may not be able to express disquiet because of deficiencies in vocabulary or lack of confidence. The learners have to be aware of and know how to deal with these different types of need.

Patients need to be able to share their anxieties with their family and friends who may be able to give practical help as well. Despite improved sick pay and National Health Insurance benefits, patients still have financial worries, particularly those with heavy hire purchase commitments and those who have to subsist on a low income even when they are well. Also, inevitably, those women with families worry about how everyone is managing in their absence, whilst professional women are concerned about their inability to meet their responsibilities at work, and students are anxious about the interruption to their studies. These patients are better provided with the means of contacting family, friends and colleagues than those of fifty years ago, there is open visiting – most essential in view of the fact that many of the visitors are on shift work – and the telephone is readily available.

The nursing staff. There are seventeen members of the nursing staff, four of whom are part-time. An increasing number of men are being accepted for training, and there is currently one male nursing student working on this ward. The following table (Table 11.1) outlines briefly some information about each nurse and gives some indication of their varied backgrounds.

You will note that eight of the staff are married and that eleven are non-resident. The fact that so many nurses are married and must give consideration to their family responsibilities has a bearing on their attitude to nursing. It is now seen in a broader context and there are advantages to this. The married, and indeed the non-resident, nurses might well have greater insight into the needs of patients than those who are protected from the stresses and strains of meeting daily responsibilities both at home and at

Table 11.1

Staff member	Age	Country of origin	Family background	Education	Resident/ Non-resident
Ward sister	25	England	Married to accountant in District Treasurer's office	Left school at 17. GCE 'O' levels 8	Non-resident
Junior sister	28	Nigeria (basic nurse training in Nigeria)	Married to law student	Left school at 18. GCE 'O' level equivalents 7	Non-resident
Staff nurse	21	England	Daughter of factory foreman	Left school at 16. GCE 'O' levels 5	Non-resident
Staff nurse Part-time	34	Wales	Married to manager of local supermarket	Left school at 15. No certificates	Non-resident
Enrolled nurse	26	Malaysia	Daughter of school teacher	Left school at 16. No GCE 'O' level equivalents	Resident
Enrolled nurse Part-time	44	England	Married to middle manager in food processing firm	Left school at 15. No certificates	Non-resident
Student nurse	20	Norway	Daughter of lawyer	Left school at 18. GCE 'O' level equivalents 6	Non-resident

(continued)

Table 11.1 (continued)

Staff member	Age	Country of origin	Family background	Education	Resident/ Non-resident
Student nurse	29	England	Son of miner	Left school at 16. GCE 'O' levels 5	Resident
Student nurse	19	England	Daughter of GP	Left school at 18. GCE 'O' levels 4 GCE 'A' levels 1	Resident
Student nurse	18	Jamaica	Daughter of bus driver	Left school at 16. GCE 'O' levels 5	Resident
Student nurse	30	England	Daughter of civil servant. Divorced – former husband owned small business	Left school at 18. GCE 'O' levels 5	Non-resident
Pupil nurse	22	Hong-Kong	Daughter of shopkeeper	Left school at 16. No GCE 'O' level equivalents	Resident
Pupil nurse	34	England	Married to senior nurse in local psychiatric hospital	Left school at 15. No certificates	Non-resident
Nursing auxilliary	25	Australia	Daughter of farmer. Working temporarily in England – seeing the world	Left school at 17. GCE 'O' level equivalents 5	Resident
Nursing auxilliary	29	England	Married to constable	Left school at 15. No certificates	Non-resident
Nursing auxilliary Part-time	48	England	Married to hospital porter	Left school at 14. No certificates	Non-resident
Nursing auxilliary Part-time	25	Italy	Married to caterer	Left school at 15. No certificates	Non-resident

work. The quality of patient care could be enhanced, always provided that these nurses are thoughtful enough to apply these insights to nursing and are sufficiently involved in their work whilst on duty.

This training school has a minimum standard of five passes in the General Certificate of Education at Ordinary level or its equivalent for student nurses, but the standard of general education of the staff as a whole is quite varied. The social and cultural backgrounds are even more varied; this is a very interesting group of people who could have much to learn from each other, given the opportunities and encouragement to do so. Notice too that part-time staff are employed, which is another indicator of the changing social scene. The profession was slow to accept part-time staff in the past but these are now usually valued members of the ward team.

Although these individuals are all so different they will be influenced to some extent by society's attitudes and values. For example, like society as a whole, the majority of nurses are unwilling to accept inadequate material rewards for their work, no matter how interesting and worthwhile it may be. Like the rest of society, nurses are influenced by those factors which lead to expectations of higher living standards. A glance at Table 11.1 will show that several of these nurses' salaries are likely to be required to supplement inadequate family incomes. In any case the majority of nurses are no longer willing to accept that they have a vocation – they generally regard nursing as a profession or a job, which, in fairness, should be rewarded like other work. Salaries and conditions of service have improved vastly since the 1930s, but increased salaries have to be considered in relation to the diminished value of money consequent on inflation. Since the introduction of the National Health Service most nurses have been employed by the State, a fact which has a bearing on salary negotiations since increased funds for improved salaries come from the public purse. However, despite some discontent over slow progress in obtaining salaries comparable with other occupational groups carrying similar responsibilities, these nurses are financially better off than their predecessors, and have longer holidays and shorter hours. Shorter hours and a higher salary provide more opportunities for cultivating interests outside nursing and for pursuing further studies. This is not to suggest that such opportunities are always recognised and used, but two nurses in this ward team are using some off-duty time to further their general education. The Malaysian Enrolled nurse is taking a course in dressmaking, and the young staff nurse is studying for GCE 'O' levels in biology and sociology.

Shorter working hours do, however, result in these nurses having less continuity of contact with patients than did their predecessors in the 1930s. This, combined with the shorter patient stay in hospital and the increased tempo of the work, leads to difficulty in the nurses getting to know individuals well enough to develop a helpful nurse/patient relationship. Similarly, because of shorter working hours, the ward sister and trained staff often have difficulty in getting to know the learners and their individual needs.

The nature of the nurses' work has changed in many respects, as was indicated at the beginning of this section when a 'bird's eye view' of ward activities was described. Other factors bringing about these changes in nursing practice will be considered in the section on advances in science and technology of particular relevance to nursing practice and education.

The learners. Perhaps it is significant that learners are no longer called probationers, a term which suggests that they are being employed on a trial basis. There are two groups of learners in this ward, student and pupil nurses. In some wards there are other groups as well, including perhaps graduates taking a shortened course for registration, post-registration or post-enrolment students taking a National Board Post Basic Course, or students taking a degree course. Relationships between individuals taking different types of course, although often excellent, may be marred by misunderstanding or jealousy; hence any hint of preferential treatment of one group by the teachers has to be avoided. The teachers, that is the trained nurses, require insight into the special needs of each group – a problem not faced by their predecessors. Different educational achievement and different life experiences are characteristic of all groups of learners wherever they may be, but in recent years nursing has attracted people of more varied cultural backgrounds than in the past, as reference to Table 11.1 will show. People in general tend to be more questioning and critical than they were in former years. Well-educated students usually expect more of their teachers, asking more difficult questions and challenging opinions as they have been taught to do at school.

These learners are still employees who are expected to provide a services as they learn from experience. Throughout the years, efforts have been made to change their status, but financial constraints, first in the voluntary and municipal hospitals and now in the National Health Service, have militated against replacing a relatively cheap labour force by more highly paid trained staff. Some of these learners are critical of their so-called student status and of the so-called apprenticeship system of nurse training. Some of their criticisms are well thought out and justified, but perhaps not all. Maybe they have received insufficient guidance about how to recognise and benefit from opportunities for learning whilst working in the clinical areas.

The developments in nursing practice have, in some respects, increased pressure on the learners, despite improvements in conditions of service and the more stringent requirements of the UKCC regarding training schemes in general and practical experience in particular. Some of the learners are more articulate than their predecessors in the 1930s and express their anxieties and dissatisfactions through staff organisations. It is worth noting evidence of the changed attitude of the profession to the expression of students' views, e.g. the establishment of the Association of Nursing Students in the Royal College of Nursing. Students now are able to exert much more influence on professional opinion than ever before. Some learners accept their wider professional responsibilities from the start of their career, and are actively involved in working for improved standards of patient care as well as for improvements in our system of nursing education.

The atmosphere of the ward is rather informal; strict discipline of the sort imposed in the 1930s would not reflect the spirit of the age and would certainly not be acceptable to the young men and women of today. Manners are more casual; this, together with the more questioning approach, has brought its tensions. Not all staff are ready to accept the challenge implicit in questioning established practices and routines, nor to take seriously suggestions and ideas put forward by learners. Some of the learners' suggestions *are* ill-founded because they may lack insight into the total situation through lack of experience, but some are good because they are able to bring a new perspective to bear on old problems. However, it is often the way in which suggestions are made or questions asked which is the root of the problem. Frequently, middle-aged staff are irritated by what they consider to be a lack of social grace and tact, and they can be misled into thinking that a brusque approach necessarily implies a lack of respect or a desire to make trouble. It is hard to adjust to changes in the social climate which, among other things, affect the way in which people speak to each other. One of the challenges faced by today's teachers is that of finding ways of helping learners to communicate effectively with people who may have very different notions of what constitutes acceptable behaviour, without sacrificing their spontaneity and sincerity. The teachers themselves require the wisdom to recognise when it is the manner rather than the matter of a learner's comments which requires correction.

The hierarchical structure of nursing persists and has perhaps been reinforced by the pattern of nursing management introduced following the implementation of the recommendations of the Salmon Committee[1] and reorganisations of the National Health Service. However, in this ward, job assignment is replaced by patient assignment so that there is less demarcation between 'senior' and 'junior' nursing tasks. Nevertheless it would be a mistake to conclude that the learners do not see some types of work as requiring more skill and knowledge, hence being 'senior' work. Sometimes their assessment of the amount of skill required for a particular task is mistaken, for reasons which will be explored further in the section on advances in science and technology of particular relevance to medicine.

The learners never attend lectures which form part of their regular training programme during their off-duty. These learners have a programme of training based on the block system and an attempt has been made to correlate theory with practice. The correlation is not perfect since allocation for practical experience has to take account of staffing needs. A clinical teacher is based in the unit, covering four wards, of which this is one. She assists the ward staff in helping the learners to benefit from their experience, liaising with the ward sister and tutors in formulating a teaching programme designed to meet the needs of individuals for guidance, support and supervision of their work in the clinical areas. A nurse tutor also works with and supervises the learners as much as possible. She and the clinical teacher are helping the ward sister to formulate learning objectives for those gaining experience in this ward.

Relaxation of hospital discipline is particularly evident when considering these learners' off-duty time. They are allowed to be non-resident after the first year of training and many elect to be so. This tends to result in less interest being shown in hospital-based social activities than there used to be. Most of the learners have sufficient resources to organise their own social functions and prefer to do so. For those who are resident, life in the nurses' home is far less supervised. They come and go pretty well as they please, the home being organised on the lines of a hostel. Wardens who have replaced the home sister are expected to see the essential rules are complied with, and to be available to the residents. The increased freedom of learners has brought its problems; these (mostly young) people have to learn to use their freedom responsibly, otherwise they may get into difficulties and their health may suffer. The teachers need to be observant to notice evidence of distress and be available to provide support in an acceptable way.

These learners may already have plans for future career development. Many opportunities are open to them now. Those who might be disadvantaged by a limited educational background can, if they want to, remedy deficiencies by attending evening classes, taking correspondence courses or perhaps studying for a degree with the Open University. There are an increasing number of post-basic clinical courses for both registered and enrolled nurses, and registered nurses also have opportunities to take advanced courses such as the Diploma in Nursing or to prepare for teaching. Since marriage no longer implies ending one's career, most of the learners are interested in finding out the possibilities for future professional development and exploring job opportunities available in this country and overseas.

The ward sister. The ward sister was appointed to her present post two years ago at the age of twenty-three – following one year's experience as a staff nurse and one year as a relief sister. She has taken a first line management course at the local technical college and a short course in examining organised by the school of nursing. Thus she had relatively limited experience of ward managment before taking up her post compared with her counterpart in the 1930s, but has had the advantage of a short introduction to management theory.

She is directly accountable to the senior nurse in the unit for the standard of nursing care in her ward. Unlike her counterpart in the 1930s, she is not responsible for planning and organising the work of the domestic staff. She does, however, have to ensure that the ward environment is suitable for patient care, which includes seeing that it is properly cleaned. To this end she liaises with the domestic superintendent and her staff. This is just one example of the present day ward sister's need to liaise with the staff of other departments contributing to patient care. Specialisation of function has developed very considerably since the 1930s, hence the work involved in co-ordinating care has become increasingly time-consuming and complex. The planning and organisation of the work of the ward team has also become morre complicated, since there is not only a larger number of team members but there are also additional constraints to be borne in mind. For example, the part-time staff work for fixed hours, which do not precisely correspond to the times of the shifts worked by full-time staff, a fact which must be allowed for when planning the off-duty. Also, when assigning responsibility for patient care, the needs of two groups of learners following different programmes of training must be considered so that each learner obtains the special experience required.

Whilst the ward sister is still an authority figure, the ward is seen to be less self-contained than it used to be since it is part of a unit, managed by the senior nurse, and part of the training school. (It always was but the implications of its being so are perhaps more clearly recognised now.) Hence, the ward sister is required to conform to agreed policies, to 'fit in' to the unit, to see that approved methods laid down by the nursing procedure committee are implemented. In short, the old ward sister tended to do things 'her way', her ward was her kingdom; the present-day ward sister is more a member of a team of managers. She is, of course, able to influence decisions and is expected to make suggestions and express opinions to her peers and seniors at unit meetings and elsewhere, e.g. she might be invited to serve on the nursing procedure committee.

The ward sister is expected to be skilled and knowledgeable in the specialised nursing undertaken in her ward. This can be a strain for the young, newly appointed ward sister who has had little opportunity to develop her own expertise before carrying the taxing responsibility of ward management. It is hard for a ward sister in this sort of situation to accept responsibility for teaching two groups of learners as well, especially if she has had no preparation for teaching. Recently, basic nurse training has included an introduction to management and teaching which should be of some help.

The ward sister in this ward is quite well equipped for her job. She is reasonably well educated, learns quickly and is a caring and committed nurse. She has had two years' experience in the ward and is universally respected; understandably, since the patients are well cared for and she has a well-integrated ward team who have been taught how to co-operate effectively with the staff of other departments. She undertakes some nursing care, working with a learner if possible, but it is difficult for her to continue giving care to a patient for any length of time without being interrupted. She practises patient assignment, believes that the nursing process provides on effective tool for delivery of nursing care, and expects each nurse to see that her particular patients receive the very best attention – she is as exacting as her predecessor of the 1930s in this regard. Sister makes sure that she observes personally and talks to all the patients by doing a ward round when she comes on duty. The round is especially necessary following her days off, since there is often a major change in the patient population during her absence.

Two consultants have beds in the ward. She is lucky in this respect since she can get to know all the doctors who care for the patients, and this is helpful in establishing good working relationships. Problems can arise in some wards where the sister works with four, five or even more teams of doctors; far too many people are involved to be able to provide for any continuity of contact between nursing and medical staff. The consultants and senior nursing staff especially need to know each other well, otherwise misunderstandings can arise all too easily. Relationships between the sister and consultants, and indeed between the patients and consultants, are less formal than in the 1930s. Special preparation is made for formal rounds, insofar as the nurse concerned sees that patients' notes and records are to hand and ensures that any equipment likely to be required is ready; but rounds are rather less impressive than they used to be.

The doctor/nurse relationship is in the process of change. Nurses are beginning to recognise and develop their own professional role and to see their contribution to patient care as involving more than carrying out treatment ordered by the medical staff. Changes in perceptions of roles and the implications of such changed perceptions, can be painful for all concerned. However, in this ward, sister is fortunate in working with medical staff who take a broad view of patient care and appreciate the extent of the contribution made by good nursing. There always have been doctors with these insights and attitudes; such doctors are likely to be among those who will be ready to accept change and who will not feel threatened by the broader concept of the nurse's role. Whatever the future holds it is vital that relationships between nurses and doctors are characterised by mutual respect and confidence, otherwise the patients will suffer. This ward sister is among those teachers who recognise that the learners need help to develop the insights and skills required to foster such relationships amid the uncertainties of change.

This ward sister has recently married and may well leave nursing for a few years whilst she has a family. She will probably expect to return to nursing, perhaps taking further courses of preparation for a senior post after resuming her career. Alternatively, she and her husband may decide not to have children – an option not open to women until recently. In this case she may continue to work as a ward sister – which she finds very rewarding, or she may consider other career opportunities outlined previously.

The changing social scene and the teacher's role

Reflection on these descriptions of the effects of social change on nursing in a women's ward in the 1930s and 1980s helps to indicate the trends which have affected patients, learners and teachers alike. It is important to recognise, however, that each individual responds in his or her own way to trends and circumstances. Generalisations about people's way of thought and life-style are useful up to a point, but can be misleading in work such as nursing, which is centred on individuals. Also, social change tends to be patchy and uneven; the total population throughout the whole country is not influenced at the same time and in the same way because circumstances differ in various geographical areas and in different sections of society.

Nevertheless, we can at this stage draw some general conclusions which have a bearing on the role of teachers in the clinical sphere.

Teachers have had to take account of changes in the learning environment. In the 1930s a well-motivated, intelligent learner in a well-run clinical area could learn a good deal from unplanned experience as a member of the caring team.

In the 1980s the increased complexity of the organisational structure, the increased interaction between staff of different departments and the accelerated pace of work have underlined the need for the formulation of learning objectives, planned experience and more support and guidance from the teachers.

Trained nurses have begun to recognise that teaching is an art and a skill for which special preparation is required. In the 1930s it seems to have been assumed that trained nurses should be able and willing to teach. Teaching in the clinical sphere was seen to comprise the provision of suitable experience insofar as this was possible, giving instruction, supervising practice and correcting faults. Now, teaching is seen to involve much more and many of those nurses teaching in the clinical sphere have received special preparation for this work.

The teachers have had to take account of changing concepts of nursing and changed perceptions of the role of the nurse. Since learners have to be taught to nurse and to fulfil the role nurses are expected to fulfil, it follows that any change in concepts of nursing or perceptions of nurses' roles must influence what the teacher teaches. For instance, if nursing now includes undertaking certain procedures not hitherto performed by nurses, then the teachers have to broaden their knowledge and learn new skills so that they are able to teach these. If nursing is seen to be more than giving routine care and carrying out medical treatment, then the teachers need to understand what else is involved, so that they can help the learners to understand as well. (See Ch. 1 and the following section.) If nurses are expected to be questioning and critical then the approach to teaching will be different from that which was appropriate when nurses were expected to conform and carry out their duties unquestioningly.

Teachers are required to take account of the changing needs of both patients and learners. In some respects human needs remain constant, but circumstances affect the health risks to which people are exposed and influence the attitudes and expectations of the patients, learners and, indeed, of the teachers themselves. Hence, if teachers in the clinical sphere are to fulfil their role successfully, it is essential that they re-appraise needs and adjust their teaching accordingly. The teachers need help to enable them to do this – a fact which underlines the importance of more adequate preparation for teaching roles.

Advances in science and technology of particular relevance to nursing practice and education

The practice of nursing is based on knowledge of physical and behavioural sciences which illuminate our understanding of the health needs of people. In the early days of this century, bodies of knowledge were certainly increasing but were relatively limited compared with those of today. Correspondingly, the relationship between knowledge of the general principles relevant to nursing care and the application of these principles to meet individual needs was relatively simple. Fewer options were open; nurses were not required to understand the principles underlying the specific management of patients suffering from a wide range of disorders, since specific medical treatment for these patients was not available at the time. There have been amazing developments in drug therapy, surgery, radiotherapy, diagnostic techniques and so on which have influenced practice in all field of nursing both in hospital and in the community. This is not to suggest that nursing was easy in the past. On the contrary, different demands were made on nursing staff in those days. Nurses required fortitude, since they needed both physical and emotional strength to look after those people for whom medical treatment was of little help. The fact that many of these people were young made particularly taxing emotional demands on the nurses. For example, it was not uncommon for young patients to die of tuberculosis as recently as the early 1940s. Good nursing care, by which was meant close observation, recognition and anticipation of the patient's needs for comfort and care, the maintenance of personal and environmental hygiene, sometimes under difficult conditions and with none of the aids available today, the maintenance of the patient's physical strength and emotional reserves through meticulous attention to his basic needs, required a great deal of skill and clinical judgement. Nursing care was seen to be of the utmost importance because, in many cases, it was all that could be offered to promote recovery.

The restricted range of knowledge and the correspondingly restricted technology meant that both nursing theory and practice was confined mainly to what we now sometimes term 'basic care'. Whilst the underlying theory was simple and, as noted above, the correlation of theory and practice was comparatively simple, the skilful application of these principles to the care of an individual was never simple. This is a point worth remembering, for it is of particular importance to teachers in the clinical sphere.

With the enormous and rapid advances in science and technology during the last few years, the theoretical basis of nursing practice has become increasingly complex; nurses have to know much more about much more in order to practise safely and intelligently. They also have to be capable of performing efficiently and safely many more skilled techniques. The profession is trying to determine the boundaries of nursing practice in a variety of specialist settings. For example, are nurse therapists *nurses*? Should nurses be expected to perform certain techniques which were formerly the province of the medical staff and, if so, in what circumstances? The correlation of theory and practice is obviously much more complex; there is a broader field of practice to be correlated with theory and more principles and facts to master in order to correlate effectively. The application of principles to the care of individuals, which was never simple, has become increasingly complicated. Learners not only

have to master much more theory but also, as always, to show
sensitivity, imagination, adaptability and empathy in their delivery
of care – which involves expressing all these qualities as well as
their intellectual understanding of needs, through their observational, interpersonal and psycho-motor skills. These considerations have a bearing on the learners' complaints about the lack of
correlation of theory and practice and on their increased awareness
of the need for support and guidance in the clinical areas.

But how much *knowledge* is required to undertake basic nursing
care safely and efficiently? Perhaps this is a non-question since it
is difficult to isolate a discrete entity 'basic nursing' – so how did
the distinction originate? The apprenticeship system of nursing
education has probably played some part in the hierarchical classification of nursing skills, as did the associated development of the
system of task allocation. Also nurses tended to up-grade skills
requiring a greater understanding of the patients' *medical* disorder
or those tasks formerly performed by doctors, rather than those
requiring the knowledge and skills of an experienced *nurse*. Hence,
when task allocation was practised, junior nurses usually performed
such basic services as sanitary rounds, bed baths and oral toilet,
whilst senior learners and qualified staff undertook the treatments,
the administration of medicines and writing of ward reports. The
position has changed and nurses question the division of care into
'basic' and 'technical' and the classification of procedures into
'senior' and 'junior' categories. Nevertheless, such ideas die hard.
Some of the patients still have the notion that it is not fitting to
ask *sister* for a bedpan, and some qualified staff still tend to believe
that certain work should not be undertaken by junior learners even
though they have had previous instruction and there is a qualified
nurse available to supervise their practice. The development of
such beliefs and attitudes shows the interaction between nursing
practice and nursing education. Where there is a limited number
of qualified staff to supervise learners' work, and where learners
constitute a large proportion of the work force, it makes sense to
provide for the patients' safety by classifying nursing tasks into
those suitable for first, second and third year learners, and seeing
that, as far as possible, the theoretical programme of instruction
matches the type of work each group is required to do. The system
always has the disadvantage of fragmenting care, to the detriment
of both patients and learners, but in recent years it has hardly been
feasible to implement. Learners in hospitals caring for the physically sick seldom nurse patients requiring full basic care who do

not also require technical nursing care. For example, bed baths are often complicated by the presence of intravenous infusions, bladder or wound drainage, and sundry other attachments which require knowledge and skill to manage safely. Both theoretical and practical teaching programmes have had to take account of such developments, for it is impossible to overlook the integration of basic and technical care in so many situations. Also, notions of 'senior' and 'junior' work can be damaging. When so-called basic care is seen to be the responsibility of the least experienced learners, it fosters the mistaken idea that basic care requires little skill. Furthermore, learners may detect insincerity in their teaching. Having been taught from the outset that giving a bedpan properly is one of the most important aspects of care, many then observe that this task is almost invariably delegated to the most inexperienced learner on duty. Insincerity is absolutely destructive of trust, engendering undesirable attitudes and cynicism in the learners, who may perhaps be forgiven for eschewing 'real' nursing in favour of more 'interesting' and less 'menial' work.

At present, much thought is being given to clarifying the concept of nursing and to identifying a body of nursing knowledge. Research into nursing practice and education is being undertaken, and nurses in this country are beginning to become more 'research minded'. It is important that all nurses should become sufficiently informed about research methods to read reports of research projects critically, so that they can judge whether the findings have relevance and application to their own field of practice. Present day teachers have the additional responsibility of ensuring that they themselves, and the learners whom they teach, are equipped to utilise research findings to the benefit of patients and future learners.

Some advances in technology have altered the face of nursing. Consider, for instance, how greatly the availability of disposables and plastic materials has modified techniques such as giving injections and performing dressings. Teachers have to be prepared to help learners and others to adapt their techniques as and when necessitated by new developments. The transition period can be difficult.

Advances in science and technology relevant to nursing practice and the teacher's role

The rapidity of changes in practice consequent on these advances has implications for both learners and teachers. The learners can be overwhelmed by too much detailed theory to the detriment of their understanding of the principles of care. New approaches to curriculum development are designed to mitigate this problem. (See Report of The Committee on Nursing. 1972.) It is recognised that post-basic nursing courses in specialised care should be developed for those who wish to study and develop skills in nursing specialties, since no nurse can expect to master the principles and practice of specialist nursing during basic training.

The teacher's role is developing in response to these needs in the following ways:

Tutorial staff are liaising more closely with nurses in the clinical areas and undertaking more teaching in these areas. Teachers in the clinical areas and tutorial staff are fnding it essential to consult together so that a coherent programme of training can be worked out. Recent developments have underlined the importance of co-operative planning, e.g. the need for clear objectives in ward-based assessments, commitments resulting from entry into the EEC, as well as the disquiet expressed by learners concerning integration of theory and practice.

Tutorial staff are tending to specialise, especially when teaching in the clinical areas. It is not possible to keep abrest of developments in *all* nursing specialities, and it is quite out of the question for teachers to become skilled in every aspect of their own field of nursing. Hence, some tutorial staff are beginning to specialise, particularly in their clinical teaching. (Specialisation poses problems which cannot be explored here, but it is suggested that the reader thinks about the pros and cons.)

An increasing number of specialist teachers are being appointed to teach post-basic nursing students. As more post-basic courses are being mounted, an increasing number of nurses who posses a teaching qualification, and who are skilled and experienced in the relevant nursing speciality, are being employed to teach registered and enrolled nurses who wish to specialise.

Nursing education: learners or workers in the clinical sphere?

Since nursing is primarily a practical art, it follows that learners' experience in the clinical sphere is of central importance, whatever the system of nursing education may be. However, the learners require a logically developed basis of theory, to which they can relate their practical experience and from which they can develop lines of enquiry and identify areas for further investigation and study. Thus, the theoretical and practical elements of any nursing course should clearly be seen to be inter-dependent and inter-related, each element providing a source of enrichment for the other. Above all, experience in the clinical areas should inspire learners to seek to perfect the application of principles of care to their practice. Hence, the quality of care in the clinical areas should be of a high standard, and sufficient guidance and support from qualified nurses with teaching skills should be available so that individual learner's needs can be identified and met. Only if all these conditions are fulfilled will learners readily perceive themselves to be learners and clinical experience be recognised as a learning experience.

How far has nursing education in this country progressed towards this ideal? For reasons explained earlier, learners, with the exception of a small minority of students taking special courses such as degree programmes, provide a service. Obviously, priority must be given to patients' needs – hence if learners constitute a high proportion of the work force their need for a particular type of experience inevitably takes second place. So provision of the appropriate experience at the appropriate stage of the course has been, and still is, a problem. As far as the quality of experience is concerned, this varies considerably despite the fact that some control is exercised by certificate awarding and examining bodies. For example, the approval of basic training schemes by the UKCC depends upon investigation into the availability of suitable clinical experience; this body is similarly concerned with the provision of suitable clinical experience for the post basic section of the English National Board. The material environment, staffing levels, the qualifications and experience of the staff, the type of experience available, and facilities for care and treatment, and as far as possible, the enthusiasm, motivation and attitudes of the staff, are all taken into account. Nevertheless, it is notoriously difficult to make objective assessments of the quality of experience, which is partly dependent on intangibles such as the commitment of staff to nursing education. Indeed, the quality of the experience is often affected by changes of personnel in the clinical areas. Furthermore, there are constraints – the statutory bodies set *minimum* standards which might be raised if the nursing service were not so dependent on the contribution made by learners.

Since dependence on learners for service gives rise to so many problems, should we aim for supernumerary learners; learners who are not members of the caring team as such but who spend a considerable part of their time practising under supervision in the clinical areas? Many leading members of the profession have thought so, and over the years committees and working parties set up to enquire into nursing education have reiterated the difficulties inherent in excessive reliance on learners as a labour force. For instance, as early as 1932 the Lancet Commission suggested that ward sisters required relief from duties to enable them to give more time to teaching. In 1938, the Athlone Inter-Departmental Committee on Nursing Services suggested – among other things, that more non-nursing staff should be employed to relieve nurses of domestic work, which would, of course, have provided more time for their learning to nurse. In 1943, the Horder Reconstruction Committee, which considered education and training, went further and recommended that schools of nursing should be independent of the hospitals providing clinical experience. The Committee did not envisage isolation of the schools from the clinical areas; on the contrary it recommended that ward sisters should be prepared for their teaching role and relieved of duties so that they would be able to undertake this important work. (The reader will remember that the country was engaged in fighting the second world war at the time.) In 1947 the Working Party on the Recruitment and Training of Nurses (chaired by Wood) made some interesting, and for that time, revolutionary recommendations for nursing education which, if implemented, would have resulted in student status for the first two years of training. This was a majority report; one member of the working party was unable to support the recommendations and produced a minority report. This suggested that further information was required and there followed a study into the work actually performed by nurses in hospital. The outcome of this study, the report on The Work of Nurses in Hospital Wards (Nuffield 1953) makes depressing reading. Among its findings are that students received almost no teaching (as little as seven minutes per week) and that, for the most part, they worked without supervision, relying on fellow students for guidance. The Platt Committee produced its report on A Reform of Nursing Education (1964) which included recommendations that schools of nursing should be independent of hospitals, that student nurses should have full student status for two years followed by a year of supervised practice, and that pupil nurse training should be planned and controlled by the school but organised on an apprenticeship basis. Finally, The Committee on Nursing (Briggs Committee 1972) produced its report. Among the

Committee's recommendations which have particular relevance here are:

1. That Colleges of Nursing and Midwifery should be established which should be independently administered, but should work in close co-operation with the practice areas;
2. That a common portal of entry to nurse training should be introduced, which would provide opportunities for all entrants to nursing to progress to more advanced studies if they so wish, provided that they have the necessary aptitudes and abilities;
3. That modular schemes of training should be planned providing:
   a. For the integration of theoretical and practical teaching;
   b. The flexibility required to build on basic modules in accordance with individual student's interests and aptitudes;
   c. The flexibility required to allow individuals to proceed to more advanced courses at their own pace and, if necessary, to resume training after a lapse of time once the basic modules had been completed.

The report emphasised the importance of close liaison between college and service staff, and suggested that for example, college staff should teach in the clinical areas and that service staff should teach in the college as and when appropriate. The profession is at the time of publication awaiting the implementation of this report.

It can be seen that for years there have been serious misgivings about the effectiveness of our present system of nursing education, and it is shortcomings in teaching in the clinical sphere which have caused most concern and comment. Some of the developments in the role of teachers in the clinical sphere should help to remedy deficiencies, but unless the learners' experience can be planned, controlled and properly supervised these developments will only serve to patch up a very ragged garment.

There has been a good deal of misunderstanding about the meaning of student status. For instance, the Platt Committee's recommendations received a very mixed reception from the profession, some nurses believing that the Committee envisaged students spending most of their time in college rather than in clinical areas. This was not so. The strength of British nursing lies in its emphasis on practical competence, but its weakness stems from a tendency to underestimate the importance of the insights derived from an understanding of the theoretical basis of practice. Many of our nurses gain these insights but they generally gain them the hard way. Such insights are essential to nurses having a supervisory role, since they must be able to see that practice is adapted to individual needs, to assign priorities, make decisions and exercise professional judgement, all of which require clinical as well as managerial expertise. We recognise this when we insist on qualified nurses managing the nursing service at all levels. Hence theory is important, perhaps more important than has hitherto been recognised, but certainly not more important than practice. Clearly, it would be impossible to teach nurses to deliver care unless they have the opportunities to practise what they are expected to learn. Planned, controlled and adequately supervised practice is the ideal we aim for, but it will not be achieved unless and until there are sufficient qualified staff available in all the clinical areas, supported by aides or auxilliary staff as the Committee on Nursing recommended.

Should the learners provide a service at all? If learners are practising nursing they inevitably make some contribution to the service. Moreover, learners not only need to practise nursing, they want to. Learners are motivated by seeing that they are actually helping patients; this is, after all, why most of them entered the profession.

There are advantages to learners working as members of the caring team. They tend to feel more accepted and probably learn more about working in co-operation with colleagues than they would as supernumerary students, contributing to the service only when undertaking certain defined responsibilities selected as part of their learning programme. Learning and working can be too sharply distinguished. In fact, learners should understand that it is always possible to learn from working with patients; if work is found to be boring and repetitious one might well ask whether the learner has forgotten about the unique characteristic of each nurse/patient interaction. The reader will recall from Chapter 1 that removing Mrs X's T-tube is a different experience from removing Mrs Y's. We can go too far in rejecting the value of working as a learning experience. It can be unwise to do so for another reason. After qualification the nurse works, and it is to be hoped that she continues to learn through working. If she believes that having completed a planned practical programme her learning is completed, she is very seriously misled.

The modular system would appear to be one way of providing the best of both worlds; practical experience is planned and integrated with theoretical work, but the learner works in the clinical area as a team member with appropriate supervision.

To sum up, both teachers in the clinical sphere and learners need to be able to identify useful learning opportunities. When learners complain that they are not taught, and when teachers complain that they have no time to teach, both groups might perhaps be overlooking the learning and teaching opportunities which exist even now. Both teaching and learning are, to some extent, dependent on an attitude of mind. The skilful teacher can help learners to see that everything they do for patients could be a learning experience. Although it is undesirable for learners to be used as 'pairs of hands', no learner worth her salt is ever just a 'pair of hands'; her head and her heart must be involved when caring for patients, so she might as well learn as much as she can from their response to her caring.

The teachers

The qualified nurses in the clinical areas

These include qualified nurses in both the hospital and the community. In principle their teaching role is similar in whatever setting they practise, but the role of the ward sister or charge nurse will receive special emphasis: firstly because the largest group of learners, those taking a basic training, spend most of their time in the wards and departments of hospitals; and secondly, because nurses in charge of the clinical areas normally have the greatest influence over the position of learning opportunities.

Has the qualified nurse's teaching role changed to any great extent over the years? Probably not in principle, but in practice it has, in some respects, become more difficult to fulfil adequately mainly because of the increased pressure on qualified staff and the decreased contact they have with learners. In addition, qualified staff in the clinical areas are members of a larger teaching team; hence there are more tutorial staff to liaise with than in the past. Finally, our concepts of teaching are broader than they were. In the early days of this century, teaching tended to be perceived as a giving of information, a supervision and direction of activities, a correction of faults. The learners' response received less attention except insofar as they were expected to take account of the teacher's directions and to work hard to achieve the standards set by the teacher. Now the teachers recognise the importance of helping learners to respond, by stimulating interest, arousing attention, fostering the motivation required for continued effort, facili tating understanding, identifying learning problems and helping learners to overcome these. Unfortunately, many qualified nurses in the clinical areas have not been taught to teach and they are not always sufficiently informed or skilled to help learners to benefit from learning opportunities.

One of the most important contributions which qualified nurses in the clinical areas can make as teachers is to see that learners gain good experience. Experience can be good in two respects. First, the experience should be of a high quality, that is, the standard of care should be excellent; secondly, the type of experience provided should be that which the learning requires. So, the qualified nurses start to fulfil their teaching role when they themselves do their own work well; that is, by providing a good role model as a skilled nurse and manager, and when they take care to allocate responsibilities to learners in accordance with each one's individual needs.

Providing a good example extends to every aspect of the qualified nurse's behaviour, including the attitudes implicit in the quality of relationships established with members of the tutorial staff. Qualified staff in the clinical areas and tutorial staff must be seen by the learners to work harmoniously together. The slightest hint of a lack of joint purpose tends to create a gulf between learning and working, the ideal and the real, theory and practice. This may tear apart the already frail links between the clinical areas and the school. Difficulties and disagreements are bound to arise from time to time but, providing all the teachers are seen to work together to resolve problems, the learners will not suffer.

In the past the sister tutor, matron and matron's assistants shared the responsibility of undertaking ward rounds. Relationships between these senior members of the staff and the ward sister tended to be very formal. Obviously, much depended on the personalities of the people involved, but the sister tutor was usually a somewhat remote figure, well-informed and a good practical nurse, judging from the comments she made during her tour of inspection. (This is how ward rounds were seen by many staff.) Now relationships are generally more informal, especially since clinical teachers and tutors actually work in the clinical areas.

The importance of the quality of the relationships between qualified nurses in the clinical areas and the tutorial staff has been emphasised so much because they must work together if the learners are to benefit from their practical experience. The qualified nurses can offer a good example, but this is only one step towards helping the learners to respond to it. The learners' response is all-important, as was pointed out at the beginning of this section. For instance, the ward sister might allow a learner to observe her interviewing a patient's relative. The ward sister listens carefully so that she can find out how she can best help the relative before giving advice, but the learner fails to observe the skill displayed in listening because her attention is directed to noticing what *advice* sister will give. Unless sister checks the learners' observations a learning opportunity will be missed. However, due to pressures of work, the sister herself may not have the time for a discussion following this experience. The tutorial staff, on the other hand, might be able to help a learner to recall and reflect on the experience and enable her to gain more from it. Of course, it would be ideal if the ward sister herself could follow through her own teaching, but sometimes compromises have to be made and the better the staff know each other the better they can co-operate. The qualified staff are often in the best position to note the individual learner's needs in the practical situation. They may have insufficient time to explore the reasons for the individual's problems let alone to deal with them, but if they themselves cannot take the necessary action they can keep the tutorial staff informed so that they can take over. Thus qualified nurses in the clinical areas should now be functioning as members of a teaching team.

Qualified nurses are now expected to be well informed about the programmes of training followed by learners gaining experience in their clinical areas, and to be involved in planning learning objectives. Representatives of the staff delivering care are usually involved in course planning, so that training schemes are designed to work well in practice. Service and tutorial staff gain a deeper insight into each other's roles and functions through working together in these ways. However, all qualified nurses require preparation for their teaching role. Some nurse managers have shown their awareness of this need by providing support and encouragement for ward sisters and charge nurses willing to take a part-time course in teaching, e.g. some have attended City and Guilds courses. Other qualified nurses have gained day-release to attend a Diploma in Nursing Course, which provides an excellent knowledge base for teaching. Many schools of nursing have provided some form of in-service training such as study days, but resources for in-service training are scarce. Following its enquiry into *Teachers of Nursing* (1975), the General Nursing Council for England and Wales set up a working party to consider the problems which had been identified. The Working Party (1975) recommended that ward sisters should attend a preparatory course in teaching to equip them for this important work. This recommendation has been echoed in the Report of the Royal College of Nursing Working Party on the Preparation and Education of Teachers of Nursing (1983).

Clinical teachers

In the late 1950s some members of the profession were of the opinion that ward sisters could no longer carry total responsibility for clinical teaching. There was a shortage or maldistribution of tutors, which meant that they were often hard pressed to fulfil their commitments in implementing the theoretical teaching programme. It might be argued that the approach to nursing education was mistaken and that tutors should not have so organised their work that they became isolated from the clinical areas, but the fact remains that more man/woman hours are required to teach nursing practice to small groups or individuals in the wards than are needed to teach a much larger group in the school. It might also be argued that more nurse tutors should have been prepared, so that tutors could undertake clinical teaching, but as usual resources were scarce and tutors are relatively expensive both to train and employ. In the event, it was decided that a new grade of nurse teacher should be introduced, and some hospitals in Scotland and in England employed clinical instructors, as they were then called.

These clinical instructors were experienced ward sisters; in some hospitals at least five years experience in the grade was required. There were seen as skilled practitioners whose sole responsibility was to support and guide learners in the clinical areas. These pioneers emphasised the importance of establishing good relationships with all the ward staff with whom they worked; they usually covered three or four wards. They had, of course, to put over their role, making it clear that they carried no responsibility for ward management, that they were not going to intrude or undermine the authority of the trained ward staff or slow down the ward work. Relationships with the tutorial staff were generally satisfactory, since it was the tutors in these schools who were among the first to see the need for clinical instructors.

The Royal College of Nursing's Education Division (as it was then) mounted courses for clinical instructors, first in Edinburgh and later in London. The Rcn course in London was requested by the General Nursing Council to accept students who intended to teach pupil nurses. Good reasons prompted this request. Firstly, many practising teachers of pupil nurses had received no preparation for their work; secondly, since the emphasis in the course for enrolment is on practical nursing, clinical teaching was seen to be of the greatest importance.

The profession did not wholeheartedly welcome clinical instructors. Some tutors feared that the introduction of a second grade of teacher – less 'well qualified' than those who had attended nurse tutor courses – would result in a lowering of standards. These fears were not without substance. Originally, clinical instructors were not envisaged as substitutes for nurse tutors but as teachers having their own special role, teaching in the clinical areas; but in fact the lack of qualified teaching staff in many schools of nursing resulted in clinical teachers undertaking work for which they had not been prepared. Furthermore, teachers of pupil nurses who attended the same course as clinical teachers generally worked in small schools in sole charge or without the support of tutors, and these teachers were responsible for nursing school administration and classroom teaching as well as for teaching in the clinical areas. This may have contributed to the poor definition of the role of clinical instructors, some teaching almost entirely in the clinical areas, some teaching partly in the classroom and partly in the clinical areas and some teaching almost full time in the classroom. Some clinical instructors became frustrated and disillusioned by this role confusion. However, some enjoyed classroom teaching and working as a clinical instructor began to be seen as the first step towards qualifying as a tutor. This notion was reinforced by the following comment in the report of the Committee on Senior Nursing Staff Structure (Salmon 1966). 'Other teaching posts in Grade 6 (Charge Nurse), those of Teacher of Pupil Nurses and Clinical Instructor, are best regarded as posts in which nurses test their aptitude for teaching before going on to become Registered Tutors. These posts entail co-operation with Ward Sisters, but prior experience as Ward Sister, as distinct from formal preparation for the job does not seem to be necessary.' (para. 7.46.). The status and position of clinical teachers, as they began to be called, vis-à-vis that the ward sister grade has always been a difficult and delicate matter. Some nurses saw teaching as an easy option with clinical teachers carrying far less responsibility than ward sisters; others pointed out that experienced ward sisters and charge nurses had undertaken a further course of training and that clinical teaching was a difficult, demanding and skilled job deserving a higher status. Confusion regarding the demands of the work and the experience required to undertake it led to some inexperienced nurses being appointed as clinical teachers, not only before appointment as a ward sister but also without formal preparation for teaching. Eventually the difficulty was, to some extent, resolved when the statutory bodies were empowered to register clinical teachers, but the requirements for registration were believed by some well-qualified clinical teachers to be disappointingly low.

Not surprisingly, in view of all this confusion, a number of clinical teachers left teaching altogether for posts offering better remuneration, status and career prospects. Some, however, were very committed teachers and stayed on despite the difficulties. Some were fortunate in working with enlightened colleagues, both in the wards and school, who appreciated how much a good clinical teacher could contribute to nursing education. Interestingly, those clinical teachers who were responsible for teaching post-certificate students attending specialist courses tended to find less difficulty than some of their 'generalist' colleagues, perhaps because their role was more clearly defined.

The General Nursing Council's enquiry into Teachers of Nursing (1975) confirmed that 33 per cent of qualified clinical teachers subsequently qualified as tutors, a wasteful process which militates against increasing the total number of teaching staff. The enquiry also uncovered some disturbing problems resulting in lack of job satisfaction, including, in some schools, poor relationships between the two grades of teacher. In view of these findings the Working Party recommended that there should, in future, be only one grade of teacher responsible for both clinical and classroom teaching. In the meantime, clinical teachers continue to be employed and nurses will seek to qualify as clinical teachers. Like all those who enjoy teaching, the real reward is the learners' response. Learners, in general, warmly welcome all who try to help them to benefit from their practical experience. The Working Party recommended that qualified clinical teachers who wish to continue to practise in that capacity should be allowed to do so, while those who would like to qualify as tutors should be offered the opportunity of applying to take an, as yet undefined, conversion course.

If the Working Party's recommendations are to be implemented to the advantage of nursing education, there must be sufficient teachers in the one grade who are capable of teaching both in the classroom and in the clinical areas. Provided that this condition is fulfilled, one can see nothing but good resulting from a move which underlines the integration of theoretical and practical teaching, but it requires the profession to change its concept of the role of the tutor. This consideration will be explored further in the next section.

Before considering the role of the tutors, it should be mentioned that nurses in the community have developed teaching roles analogous to that of the clinical teacher. Fieldwork teachers supervise and guide student health visitors' practice, whilst practical work teachers perform the same function for students preparing for a qualification in district nursing. The establishment of these grades of teacher is another indication of growth in the area of post-certificate teaching in the clinical sphere.

The tutors

For many years tutors in hospital were based mainly in the classroom. This was understandable since there has always been a paucity of resources for nursing education, and the ratio of learners to tutors was high. Also the reader will recall that the theoretical programme of training has had to develop in response to advances in knowledge. The study day and block release systems were introduced to provide time for learners to be presented with ever-increasing amounts of theory, and demands on the tutors were correspondingly increased. Then, as noted earlier, there was also a tendency to see teachers as people who gave lectures, set and marked written work and so on. This concept of a teacher was attractive to some nurses who genuinely enjoyed 'imparting knowledge'. A few nurses saw teaching as an escape from the pressures of patient care and ward management, and some senior staff saw teaching as suitable work for nurses who were not physically robust. Note that yet again teaching was considered by some to be an easy option. Whilst it is true that classroom teaching requires less physical stamina than ward work, clinical teaching in general wards is often found to be more physically tiring than the work of a ward sister, since the teacher can be involved in heavy nursing care for most of the day.

It is important to bear these considerations in mind when thinking about the developing role of tutors in the clinical sphere. We have to start from where we are – there are some experienced tutors who, for various reasons may be unable or unwilling to undertake much clinical teaching. Added to these problems there is the fact that some tutors, who have not been teaching in the clinical areas, may find it difficult to get in touch again and, of course, those who took the tutor's course some years ago have had no specific preparation for teaching in the clinical areas. Furthermore, clinical teaching usually involves one-to-one or small group teaching – a fact which implies that we must improve our current teacher/learner ratio. It will also be essential to utilise fully the teaching skills of all the qualified nurses in the clinical areas.

These are the problems which the profession, and particularly the tutors, must face and resolve when there is only one grade of nurse teacher responsible for both classroom and clinical teaching. Nevertheless, many tutors are enthusiastic about teaching in the clinical areas and have increasingly incorporated more clinical teaching in their own teaching programmes. They are well aware that any attempt to make a sharp division between teaching nursing theory and practice is an expedient. It is always an artificial division and is obviously an impediment to the aim of helping learners to integrate theory and practice. After all, if Mr A teaches the theory of nursing a patient suffering from renal failure on Tuesday, and Miss B teaches the practice on Thursday, there is a natural tendency for learners to separate these learning experiences, despite their teachers' efforts to forge links between these sessions. It is also an advantage that some tutors have received special preparation for clinical teaching, those who qualified as clinical teachers before taking the tutor's course. A proportion of these are very committed clinical teachers who, possibly because of family responsibilities, took a further qualification to improve their career prospects. Students recently taking tutor's courses will have been encouraged to see themselves in the 'new' tutor's role, and since the vast majority miss the satisfaction derived from involvement in patient care when they first take up teaching, they are likely to welcome the prospect of teaching where patients are being nursed.

If all the nurses teaching in the clinical sphere can learn to work together effectively, and if they all receive proper preparation for their teaching roles, then the future of nursing education could be bright. We are developing insights into the needs; now we have to work out precisely how we intend to put our ideas into practice and to unite in pressing for the resources which are essential to translate the vision into reality.

REFERENCES

Briggs (1972) Report of the Committee on Nursing. London: M.M.S.O.
General Nursing Council for England and Wales (1975) *Teachers of Nursing.*
General Nursing Council for England and Wales (1975) Report of the Working Party on Teachers of Nursing.
Goddard, H. A. (1953) *The Work of Nurses in Hospital Wards.* Nuffield.
Platt Report (1964) *A Reform of Nursing Education.* London: Royal College of Nursing.
Report of the R.C.N. Working Party (1983) *The Preparation and Education of Teachers of Nursing.* London: Royal College of Nursing.
Salmon (1966) Report of the Committee on Senior Nursing Staff Structure, London: H.M.S.O.

FURTHER READING

Baly, Monica E. (1980) *Nursing and Social Change,* 2nd edn. London: Heinemann.
Hollingworth, S. (1985) *Preparation for Change.* London: Royal College of Nursing.

Glossary

Affective domain	The feeling and emotional aspect of experience.
Affiliation	The feeling of 'belongingness' – of attachment to another or others.
Aim	A foreseen end that can be used to give direction to an activity or to motivate behaviour – a long-term goal.
Anxiety	A complex emotional state with apprehension or dread as its most prominent component which has physiological signs associated with activity of the sympathetic nervous system.
Apprenticeship system of training	The traditional method of nurse training in the U.K. where the learner does not have full student status, and where the skills of nursing are learned largely 'on the job', under instruction from the employer, for a specified period of time.
Assessment	An estimate of the effectiveness of learning, or teaching. Can be carried out by the individual himself or by the teacher.
Assessment (continuous)	A form of student evaluation where *every* piece of work which the student performs or produces throughout the course is appraised. Not to be confused with intermittent assessment where *a set number* of pieces of work throughout the course are appraised. These systems may or may not be used in association with formal examination methods of assessment.
Associative learning	Emphasises mechanical connections and associations between events. When two or more inputs of information are received by the perceptual systems at approximately the same time, any property that one may have for eliciting action is acquired by the other; the two inputs or stimuli become associated.
Attention	The selective activity characteristic of the mental life. In teaching the term can be interpreted loosely as *concentration* and thus it depends upon the student's level of arousal and motivation.
Attitude	A more or less stable set or disposition of opinion, interest or purpose, involving expectancy of a certain kind of experience and readiness with an appropriate response.

Body image	The individual's unique perception of his own physical being.
Chaining	A sequential form of organisation, where one stage is linked to the next. May be hierarchical, a simple series, a chain of causes and effect, etc.
Clinical field	Used here to refer to wherever the patient, or potential patient, *is*, i.e. it is not restricted to the narrow sense of 'at the bedside'.
Clinical judgement	The ability to make professionally appropriate decisions on nursing care. Such judgement is developed through professional education and practice and rests on a range of skills, both technical and caring, in the areas of perception, selection, assessment, intervention and evaluation.
Clinical nurse specialist	A practising nurse of some seniority who has specialised in a particular branch of nursing (e.g. stoma therapy) and who is called upon to give nursing advice to both patients and nursing staff over the hospital and community area in her particular field of expertise.
Cognition theories	A collective term for the theories pertaining to the psychological processes involved in the acquisition, organisation and use of knowledge.
Cognitive domain	The knowing, perceiving, conceiving aspect of experience, as opposed to emotion and volition (see affective domain).
Communication	A process by which people influence one another by transmitting and receiving ideas, opinions, feelings and attitudes, usually involving the use of language. Whether what is received is the same as what is transmitted therefore depends on a common perception of the meanings of the language or symbols used.
Communication, non-verbal	The larger interpersonal context within which all verbal communications take place. All human actions are suffused with meaning, and one's facial expressions, posture, gestures, etc., convey meanings which may enhance or modify one's verbal discourse. Such actions provide clues for interpreting the meaning of verbal language.
Concepts	The idea of a class of objects. The meaning of a term and thus the smallest unit of thought. Concepts combine to form propositions or complete thoughts. To acquire a concept is primarily to learn, and to possess a concept is primarily to know.
Conditioning (classical)	The process by which a response comes to be elicited by a stimulus, object or situation other than that to which it is the natural or normal response.
	Originally used for the case in which a reflex normally following on stimulus A comes to be elicited by a different stimulus B, through the constant association of B with A.

Conditioning (operant) (also known as instrumental conditioning)	A form of conditioning in which behaviour is controlled through systematic manipulation of the consequences of previous behaviour. Reinforcement is central to the process. Knowledge of (or control over) the delivery of reinforcements in a given situation is both a necessary and sufficient condition for the prediction or control of behaviour.
Consolidation	The joining together of units of learning into a cohesive whole. For consolidation to occur, the student requires time to go over the subject matter after the initial presentation, repetition and revision.
Counselling	A process through which one person helps another by purposeful conversation in an understanding atmosphere. It seeks to establish a helping relationship in which the one counselled can express his thoughts and feelings in such a way as to clarify his own situation, come to terms with some new experience, see his difficulty more objectively and so face his problems with less anxiety and tension. Its basic purpose is to direct the individual to make his own decision from among the choices available.
Crisis teaching	Teaching about things as they happen, without benefit of planning or prior knowledge of what will occur, as in the ward where the clinical teacher guides the student through sudden changes in patient management necessitated by the patient's critical condition.
Curriculum	A specified course of study.
Deductive learning	Learning by arguing from the general to the particular (see inductive learning).
Defense mechanisms	Involuntary or unconscious measures adopted by an individual to protect himself against the painful affect associated with some highly disagreeable situation, physical or mental.
Demonstration	A carefully prepared presentation that shows how to perform an act or use a procedure.
Discovery learning	A system of learning in which the student is presented with a problem and the tools with which to find the solution to the problem, and proceeds with a varying degree of guidance to discover for himself or herself the theory on which the solution rests.
Feedback	Knowledge of results. The sooner it is acquired, after testing, the more effective it is. May be verbal or non-verbal.
Gestalt psychology	Originated in Germany in the early 20th century as a psychology of perception. 'Gestalt' means pattern, configuration or organised whole with qualities different from those of its components separately considered – e.g. a melody.
Halo effect	A tendency to be biased in the estimation or rating of an individual with respect to a certain characteristic, by some irrelevant impression or estimate (good or bad) of the same individual.

Hardware	In computer technology, the term refers to the actual computer or associated gadgetry. Used here more loosely to refer to the machinery or equipment used as teaching aids.
Inductive learning	Learning by drawing general conclusions from particular instances (see deductive learning).
Item bank	A collection of valid questions for use and re-use in objective test-type assessments, covering a syllabus or an area of a syllabus.
Lateral thinking	Aims to bypass obstacles in a chosen line of approach to the solution of a problem by switching to radically different approaches involving a reformulation of the problem.
Learning resource centre	An area in which are gathered together systems or vehicles for the transmission of information – e.g. library, visual-aids centre.
Media resources officer	An expert conversant in the use of learning resources – i.e. methods for the transmission of information.
Microfiche (ERIC)	A device which allows large amounts of information to be stored in a small space. A transparent card with several pages of print microscopically printed on it is inserted into a microfiche reader, the correct page is selected and the reader then magnifies the page and allows the information to be read off.
Modular system	A system (used here in relation to nurse training) in which the matter to be learned is broken down into discrete units and practice follows immediately upon the learning of the theory, with a consolidation period following on from the practice.
Mores	Term applied to a social group covering, over and above the recognised principles of conduct, those laws and customs regarded as essential and vital to the group (e.g. 'Thou shall not kill').
Motivation	The force which energises and gives direction to behaviour. Motivation may be increased by the desire for relevance, curiosity, enthusiasm from the teacher, the need for social interaction, achievement drive, fear, the need for esteem.
Need	A condition marked by the feeling of lack or want of something, or of requiring the performance of some action. Needs may motivate behaviour, e.g. lack of food motivates the hungry person to seek nourishment.
Negative learning	Learning how to do something by experiencing first how *not* to do it, e.g. one could learn points about how to teach from suffering under a poor teacher who fails to interact with students, delays feedback, etc.
Nightingale ward	The traditional arrangement for a hospital ward up to about 1960, with unpartitioned beds situated regularly up either side of a rectangular area. More recently, beds are arranged in wards in bays, or single or four to six bedded rooms.

Norms	Two usages are common: (1) What is normal or usual behaviour in some community or social group. (2) An ideal or standard to which people think behaviour ought to conform, or which some legislating authority lays down. The two may coincide but frequently they differ.
Nursing diagnosis	The formulation of a patient's nursing problems. These may differ from the medical diagnosis, although they may be consequent upon it. There may be several nursing diagnoses, e.g. a patient 24 hours after a spinal fusion may have the following nursing diagnoses: 1. difficulty in feeding and drinking 2. difficulty in micturition 3. difficulty in seeing what is going on 4. potential for developing pressure sores and fear of moving
Nursing history	The information obtained from whatever source (the patient, relative, records, etc.) pertaining to the nursing care of the patient during his stay in hospital. Usually obtained in interview with the patient. Information sought is that on which assessment can take place in order to plan care.
Nursing process	A dynamic problem-solving approach to nursing which seeks to individualise care. Essentially consists of four stages: 1. *Assessment*. The patient's needs are sought and relevant information is brought to light that may have a bearing upon the patient's care. 2. *Planning*. A care plan is drawn up in accordance with the patient's perceived needs. 3. *Implementation* (or intervention). The delivery of care. 4. *Evaluation*. The care given is assessed for its value to the patient in the light of assessment.
Objective	A specific, measurable, behavioural end that the learners are trying to reach, i.e. what the learners should be able to do at the end of the teaching. Often referred to as behavioural or instructional objectives.
Objective tests	Tests in which the questions are so presented that there can be only one correct response or set of responses, and the examiner's own interpretation is eliminated from the marking process. The instructions and time allowed are standardised and usually such tests are made up of a battery of subjects. A *multiple choice* test is one version of an objective test.
Observation	Careful and attentive examination of phenomena with a view to a clearer knowledge.
One-to-one learning	The ideal situation where there is one teacher to every single learner. Clinical teachers work frequently in this way, more because of the nature of their work than because of an abundance of manpower. This method is obviously expensive on teaching time.

Overteaching	The tendency to teach more, and in greater depth, than is required by the aims and objectives of the teaching session. Occurs frequently when the teacher has not specified her objectives clearly and realistically.
Patient allocation	A system of organising nursing care where individual nurses are responsibile for the total care of individual patients. Also called total patient care or patient-centred care.
Perception	In general, awareness or appreciation of objects or situations, usually by the senses. The way in which we perceive objects is influenced by our past experience, e.g. a trained nurse on a train may notice signs and symptoms in other passengers that would escape the uninitiated. A degree of subconscious selection occurs. Therefore, in our everyday perception, factors which are irrelevant to our state of learning or past experience are filtered out.
Post-test	A test – normally objective – given after a piece of teaching to assess its effectiveness. Usually given in conjunction with a pre-test.
Prejudice	Literally 'to prejudge'. A relatively enduring attitude normally with emotional aspects, hostile to (or in favour of) actions or objects of a certain kind, certain factors or certain doctrines. Resistant to appeals to logic.
Pre-test	A test – usually objective – given before a teaching session to ascertain the student's state of knowledge. Thus, if a post-test is used, the amount of learning that has taken place can be measured. Some form of pre-test, however sketchy or informal, is necessary if one is to move 'from the known to the unknown' and 'start off where the student is'.
Problem-solving approach	The form of activity where the organism is faced with a goal to be reached, a gap in the route to the goal and a set of alternative means of reaching the goal. This forms an approach to nursing care whereby the problem is formulated in the nursing diagnosis, the planning stage is the decision-making stage and the evaluation stage estimates the degree to which the nursing problem has been solved.
Programmed texts	Books in which the material to be learned is presented in an order and form which is designed to make learning easy and to bring out the interconnectedness of the subject manner. The material is broken into small steps (frames) with a precise objective for each frame. After completing a frame the reader has to answer a question unit. If he makes a correct response he can proceed to the next frame. Thus he obtains immediate feedback on his learning. Pre- and post-tests are frequently incorporated into these texts.
Psychomotor domain	Refers to the movements, and thus skills, induced by mental processes.

Rapport	A relationship based on a high degree of community of thought, interest and sentiment.
Readiness to learn	Having the prerequisites for learning (e.g. one has a readiness to learn the nursing management of nephrotic syndrome when one possesses a knowledge of the physiology of the renal tract and the appropriate pathology of the condition).
Reception learning	A passive form of learning where the student receives the information purveyed largely without question and 'plays back' this material to the teacher in its original form.
Reinforcement	This may be negative as well as positive. A positive reinforcer, according to the psychologist B. F. Skinner, is a stimulus that strengthens the probability of a response when it is added to a situation (i.e. it is a reward for a correct response). A negative reinforcer is one that strengthens response probability when it is removed from the situation (i.e. it is a punishment for an incorrect response).
Role	Connotes the bundle of formal and predictable attributes associated with a particular social position, as distinct from the personal characteristics of the individual who occupies that position. Officially and publicly recognised roles such as that of doctor or nurse are supported by uniforms and strict linguistic codes. Most social roles, however, are not so exactly defined.
Role expectations	That which is expected of the holder of a particular role by other members of the in-group or reference group or by the public, e.g. a role expectation of a nurse is that she should be kind and gentle. Conflict ensues when the role expectations are not fulfilled.
Role model	A person who fulfils a role such that she provides an example for those who are aspiring to occupy the role, e.g. a clinical teacher provides a role model for the student nurse.
Role play	Situation where students are given certain social roles and freely dramatise them in a group, i.e. they act out their specified roles. Primary objectives of this method include development of empathy, self-awareness, attitude-change and the working-off of tensions.
Rote learning	Learning by heart, by repetition, with little or no understanding.
Self-actualisation	The process by which an individual comes to understand his own strengths and weaknesses and thereby develops his talents and capacities with acceptance of his limitations.
Seminar	A group discussion introduced by the presentation of an essay or other work. Primary objectives for this method include the development of critical thinking, thought at all levels and the ability to present an argument.

Set	The development of a 'learning set' results from solving large numbers of problems, and the skill developed represents strategies useful in solving new problems within the same general category. It is therefore a predisposition to learn a certain thing in a certain way and involves transferring previously learned skills to a new situation.
Shaping behaviour	A mechanism involved in the development of new responses in which behaviour is slowly modified by the use of reinforcers. The behaviour is therefore controlled externally by a carefully designed programme of rewards or punishment until the desired response is obtained.
Sign learning	The student makes diffuse responses to signals in the environment, e.g. as the reflex responses of the baby are triggered by an increasing number of stimuli, the baby comes to learn that certain events come to *signal* other kinds of events, as when being picked up becomes a signal for eating, and the baby thus learns to respond appropriately.
Skills	May be either a physical or mental performance of anything that a person has learned to do with ease and precision. The learning process that led to this high degree of performance has become internalised such that the skill requires little thought for its performance, i.e. it is automatic.
Socialisation	The induction of an individual into a culture's values, rules and ways of operating, so that he will be accepted by society and will become a recognised, co-operative and efficient member of it.
Software	In computer technology, this refers to the programs, as distinct from the hardware, of the computer; as it is used here, it refers to the materials necessary for the functioning of the machine, e.g. the software for an overhead projector would be the acetate sheets and frames.
Stimulus-response learning	The type of learning that is acquired with classical or operant conditioning.
Structured teaching	A planned approach to teaching where the session has a definite format usually imposed by the teacher. Structured teaching by the clinical teacher may have to give way to crisis teaching, where the session is unplanned and the boundaries are set by the crisis or emergency as it occurs. Completely unstructured teaching, where no guidance is given to the learner, is not a common strategy in nurse training.
Subjective judgements	Judgements resting on the individual's introspective data. In the formation of such judgements, there is little or no appeal to objective, rational data and they may thus be prejudiced. Halo effects may distort the resultant estimation.

Objective judgement aims to remove all subjective elements and to be based on a rational, logical assessment.

Status
Used to describe different social evaluations – in the form of rank, prestige etc. – of a person or group. Status distinctions may be marked by differences in life-styles, power, etc.

Stereotype
An oversimplified mental image of some category of person, institution or event which is shared, in essential features, by large numbers of people. Stereotypes are commonly, but not necessarily, accompanied by prejudice.

Syllabus
An abstract which gives headings or main subjects of a course of teaching, a programme of hours of work.

Systems analysis
This is a computer term. A system is a group of related elements organised for a purpose. Systems analysis consists of analysing a whole task in its setting and deciding in outline how to arrange it for the computer; estimating how much work is involved; dividing the process into a number of relatively independant parts; and finally specifying each of these, together with their interconnections.

Systems model of teaching
The analysis of the teaching process into a sequence of logical steps, akin to those used in the nursing process. The steps used are:
1. analysis of task
2. assessment of student potential
3. setting of objectives
4. selection of methods and resources
5. delivery of teaching
6. testing of achievement of objectives
7. evaluating the teaching

Task allocation
A system of organising nursing care in which each nurse is responsible for performing a particular task for every patient on the ward who requires it, e.g. one nurse may carry out all the dressings, another may collect all the specimens, etc. Also called job allocation, task- or procedure-orientated care.

Task analysis
The breakdown of a task or skill into its minutest constituent parts for the purpose of teaching the skill. It ensure that the learner masters each small step along the way to internalising the total skill.

Taxonomy
A classification scheme.

Team nursing
A way of organising nursing care in which a team of nurses collectively looks after a group of patients. The team consists of a senior team leader, who co-ordinates the care, and junior members, who deliver care under supervision. This form of nursing is a movement towards total patient care.

Team teaching	Teaching performed by a team of teachers responsible for a group of pupils. A team teaching session on renal failure might involve the clinical teacher, the dietician, the medical social worker and the doctor. Each member contributes to the total plan in accordance with her particular area of expertise.
Total patient care	The system of nursing in which the total care of each patient is assigned to a particular nurse. Each patient has 'his own' nurse. The delivery of total patient care is enhanced by the use of the nursing process. (see also patient allocation).
Trial and error learning	A type of learning most characteristically shown in animals. Learning is marked by the successive trial of various responses to a situation, ostensibly at random, until one is successful and attains the goal.
Tutorial group	Learning situation in which the topic and general direction of the session are given by the teacher, but the context and direction of the discussion depend on the student group. It develops understanding and thinking at all levels.
Tutorial, individual	A period of teaching devoted to a single student. It encourages individual development of student thought, especially at higher levels (see one-to-one learning).
Validity	The extent to which a test measures that which it is intended or purports to measure.
Value judgement	An utterance which asserts or implies that some thing, person or situation is good or bad, or some action ought or ought not to be done.
Ward learning programme	A plan drawn up of all the possible learning opportunities that learners may encounter on a particular ward, together with the appropriate objectives. These are largely ward-specific.
Worksheet	A handout that can be given to a student at the start of a ward experience or workshop for her to work through, using suitable references, and to complete by the end of her time on the ward or workshop. The student is frequently asked to define terms, plan care, assess priorities, etc., and therefore objectives must be carefully set before the worksheet is devised. May also be called a workbook.
Workshop	A contrived learning setting which offers opportunities for students with a common interest or problem to meet with specialists, or to have access to relevant resources, in order to learn.

Index